LASERS IN OTOLARYNGOLOGY

Lasers in Medicine and Surgery Series

General Editors

Mr J. A. S. Carruth,
Department of Otolaryngology,
Royal South Hants Hospital,
Southampton, UK.

Professor S. N. Joffe,
College of Medicine,
University of Cincinnati Medical Center,
Cincinnati,
Ohio, USA

Lasers are finding increasing uses in many branches of medicine and surgery. This new series will review the applications in various specialities, and will provide authoritative and up to date accounts of current practice. Each editor will select an international team of contributors chosen for their particular expertise. Little background knowledge of lasers will be assumed, and the books should therefore appeal to all physicians and surgeons in the relevant speciality.

LASERS IN OTOLARYNGOLOGY

Edited by

J. A. S. Carruth
and
G. T. Simpson

CHAPMAN AND HALL

First published in 1988 by
Chapman and Hall Ltd
11 New Fetter Lane, London EC4P 4EE

© 1988 Chapman and Hall Ltd

Printed in Great Britain at the
University Press, Cambridge

ISBN 0 412 30940 8

All rights reserved. No part of this book may be
reprinted, or reproduced or utilized in any form or
by any electronic, mechanical or other means,
now known or hereafter invented including
photocopying and recording, or in any information
storage and retrieval system, without permission
in writing from the publisher.

British Library Cataloguing in Publication Data

Lasers in otolaryngology.—(Lasers in
medicine and surgery).
1. Otolaryngology. Use of lasers
I. Carruth, J.A.S. II. Simpson, G.T.
III. Series
616.2'2'0028

ISBN 0-412-30940-8

1 Contents

	Contributors	ix
	Preface	xi
1.	Lasers – physics, tissue interaction and safety ALAN L. McKENZIE	1
1.1	Laser physics	1
1.2	Laser–tissue interaction	19
1.3	Laser safety	24
	References	31
	Further reading	31
2.	Anaesthesia for CO_2 laser surgery A. C. WAINWRIGHT	35
2.1	The surgical requirements	35
2.2	The surgical stimulus	35
2.3	General health of adult patients	35
2.4	Complications of the CO_2 laser	36
2.5	Techniques with adults	37
2.6	Patients with a tracheostomy	43
2.7	Lesions in the mouth	43
2.8	Paediatric patients	44
	References	44
3.	The laser in laryngeal disease GEORGE T. SIMPSON	47
3.1	Introduction	47
3.2	Anaesthesia	48
3.3	Exposure of the operating field	48
3.4	Adequate time for unhurried surgery	50
3.5	Magnification	50
3.6	Special instruments	50
3.7	Safety	51
3.8	Postoperative care	53
3.9	Major surgery for specific benign organic lesions	54

3.10	Premalignant and malignant disease	72
3.11	Summary	84
	References	85

4.	Endoscopic laser surgery of the tracheobronchial tree	87
	GRAEME A. McDONALD and M. STUART STRONG	
4.1	The CO_2 laser system	87
4.2	Nd-YAG laser system	93
4.3	Soft tissue interaction	94
4.4	Interactions	95
4.5	Contraindications	96
4.6	Pre-operative and postoperative evaluation	96
4.7	Complications	97
4.8	Discussion	98
4.9	Summary	99
	References	99

5.	CO_2 laser surgery in the oral cavity	101
	P. H. RHYS EVANS and J. W. FRAME	
5.1	Alternative surgical techniques: uses and limitations	101
5.2	The CO_2 laser: advantages	102
5.3	Use of the CO_2 laser in the mouth	102
5.4	Healing of laser wounds of oral mucosa	109
5.5	Anaesthetic and safety aspects: special considerations in the oral cavity	114
5.6	Treatment of oral lesions	114
5.7	Complications of CO_2 laser surgery	128
	References	131

6.	Micro-endoscopic CO_2 laser surgery of the hypopharyngeal diverticulum	133
	J. J. M. VAN OVERBEEK	
6.1	Aetiology, symptoms and diagnosis	133
6.2	Therapy	134
6.3	Discussion	142
	References	144

7.	The role of lasers in nasal surgery	147
	A. P. BRIGHTWELL	
7.1	The CO_2 laser	147
7.2	The argon laser	148
7.3	The Nd-YAG laser	149
7.4	Laser technique	149
7.5	Laser applications in the nose	152
	References	155

8.	The use of the laser in otology	157
	J. J. PHILLIPPS	
8.1	Experimental background	157
8.2	Clinical applications	160
8.3	External ear and external auditory meatus	160
8.4	Tympanic membrane and middle ear	161
8.5	Acoustic neuroma	164
	References	165
9.	Photodynamic therapy	167
	J. CARRUTH	
9.1	Tumour sensitizer	167
9.2	Light sources	170
9.3	Animal studies	171
9.4	Clinical studies	171
9.5	Conclusion	173
	References	174
	Index	177

1 Contributors

A. P. BRIGHTWELL FRCS
Otolaryngologist, Southampton Laser Unit and Southampton University Hospitals, UK

J. A. S. CARRUTH FRCS
Otolaryngologist, Southampton Laser Unit and Southampton University Hospitals, UK

J. W. FRAME PhD, FDSRCS
Reader in Oral Surgery, Birmingham University. Consultant in Oral Surgery, Birmingham University Hospitals, UK

G. A. McDONALD FACS, FRCSC
Department of Otolaryngology, Boston University School of Medicine, Boston, MA, USA

A. L. McKENZIE PhD
Principal Physicist, Newcastle General Hospital, Newcastle-upon-Tyne, UK

J. J. PHILLIPPS FRCS
Otolaryngologist, Southampton Laser Unit and Southampton University Hospitals, UK

P. H. RHYS EVANS DCC, FRCS
Director of the Head and Neck Unit, The Royal Marsden Hospital, London, UK

G. T. SIMPSON MD, MPh, FACS
Associate Professor of Otolaryngology, Boston University Medical Center, Boston, MA, USA

M. STUART STRONG MD, FACS
Department of Otolaryngology, Boston University School of Medicine, Boston, MA, USA

J. J. M. VAN OVERBEEK MD
ENT Department, University Hospital and Deaconess Hospital, Gronigen, The Netherlands

A. C. WAINWRIGHT FFARCS
Consultant Anaesthetist, Southampton University Hospitals, UK

Preface

Albert Einstein described the basic physics of stimulated emission of radiation in 1917 but it was not until 1960 that the first laser was produced by T. H. Maiman using a synthetic ruby as the lasing medium.

Since then, a vast number of lasers have been developed producing both pulsed and continuous wave coherent light in all parts of the visible and invisible spectrum. The range of uses of these lasers is now so great and so diverse that it has been suggested that the age in which we live will eventually become known as the laser age rather than either the atomic or space age.

As each laser was developed its effects on body tissues were investigated. In the case of the carbon dioxide laser, which is now the most commonly used laser in otolaryngology, this involved moving the experimental animals on moveable tables beneath the fixed, laboratory bench laser.

However, from the mid 1960s using rather more sophisticated and clinically orientated machines, a considerable amount of research took place on the effects of this laser on a wide range of tissues and its potential value as a 'light scalpel' became apparent.

Much of the credit for the introduction of the carbon dioxide laser into otolaryngology must go to the 'Boston group'. Here a unique and imaginative team of physicists, scientists, instrument makers and surgeons collaborated to define the effects of this laser on laryngeal tissues, first in animals and subsequently in man. They then developed appropriate delivery systems and endoscopes to enable clinical work to begin.

This group identified at an early stage the need for all these workers to collaborate to ensure that laser tissue interactions were fully understood and then translated into clinical practice using appropriate machines and delivery systems. This model has become the standard for all other laser units developed throughout the world.

In 1971, Dr. Stuart Strong and Dr. Geza Jako began the first clinical studies in man and following the development of other laser systems, within America and throughout the world, the use of the carbon dioxide laser escalated in this field and its value has now become fully established.

Preface

At present the infrared coherent laser beam cannot be transmitted via a flexible fibre and a hollow articulated arm with mirrors at the angles must still be used. However, it seems certain that a fine diameter efficient fibre will soon be available for use with this laser.

Another interesting and potentially important development with the continuous wave carbon dioxide laser is the introduction of super pulsing of the beam with high peak power and short exposure. Theoretically, and in practice, this results in instantaneous vaporization of tissue with less charring and with less thermal damage to adjacent tissues. There is a small but relatively insignificant loss of haemostasis but time will show if the reduction of tissue reaction will result in a further reduction in the contracture of laser wounds, and if this proves to be the case then it should be possible to achieve better results than at present in the laser treatment of laryngeal stenosis. Future developments will depend on the physicists and scientists defining exactly the tissue response to lasers of different wavelengths with various powers and exposures and surgeons will then marry this information to their clinical needs and laser manufacturers will produce machines capable of delivering the appropriate treatment parameters. It has been said that the laser surgeon must become a 'biomedical engineer' and although this remains true, few if any surgeons can acquire the laboratory expertise to perform both the experimental and clinical work and collaborative groups are essential.

However, in all medical laser applications the words of Dr. Leon Goldman, one of the fathers of laser surgery, must never be forgotten, 'If you don't need the laser, don't use it'. A laser should only be used when it can perform a particular task better than existing conventional techniques. The carbon dioxide laser has proved its worth in otolaryngology, especially in microlaryngeal surgery particularly on children. The evidence for the value of the argon laser in otology is increasing but at present the case for its use remains 'unproven'. The Neodymium YAG laser has established its role in endobronchial surgery and it will be interesting to compare this laser with the carbon dioxide laser in this field, especially when a delivery fibre is available for the infrared carbon dioxide laser beam.

Photodynamic therapy represents a new and exciting modality for the treatment of many forms of malignant disease. A photosensitive tumour localising drug is given and then activated within the tumour by laser light of the appropriate wavelength. Using haematoporphyrin derivative and red laser light produced by either a tunable dye or gold vapour laser, some exciting preliminary results are being obtained. The head and neck tumour is particularly suitable for this form of treatment

Preface

as it is relatively small, accessible, metastasises late and surgery is always mutilating to either the appearance of patients or to their ability to talk and swallow. Within this field control of some advanced lesions has been achieved, and a 'cure' with a follow-up of more than two years in a small number of patients with early lesions, who were unsuitable for other treatment modalities.

It is not difficult to learn to use a laser attached to the operating microscope but it is difficult to use it well. Safety is of the utmost importance and the establishment of required training standards for doctors before using medical lasers, remains a thorny and unsolved problem on both sides of the Atlantic.

Before beginning work with a surgical laser the surgeon must ensure that the machine conforms to all the appropriate national and international standards and that all national and local codes of safe practice are being followed to the letter. The surgeon should also have spent time studying the techniques 'at the feet of an established master' and ideally should have a chance to develop them on the cadaver or experimental animal.

Before beginning clinical work, a team must be formed with one or more anaesthetists who are fully conversant with the hazards of laser anaesthesia and how to overcome them.

Few additional instruments beyond those normally provided for microlaryngeal surgery will be needed, but the surgeon must be fully conversant with the absorptive and reflective properties of the materials from which the instruments are made. He must also ensure that there is no excessive absorption with heating of the instrument, and that surfaces from which the beam could be reflected back into the operating theatre are roughened to ensure that any reflection is diffuse.

It is vitally important to suck away the vapour produced by tissue destruction at the point of surgery, both for visual access and to ensure that the steam does not damage normal tissues. A wide range of suction devices are available which can be attached to the laryngoscope or are combined with mirrors, retractors or microlaryngeal forceps to ensure that adequate suction can be provided in all operative situations.

In the past it has been stated that a lesion has been removed using the carbon dioxide laser but in future this information must be combined with details of the exact excision parameters, including power, power density, fluence etc. In this way optimal treatment parameters for each clinical condition will eventually be defined.

The authors in this volume combine the best from both sides of the Atlantic. This book represents a state of the art account of the current use of lasers in all fields within otolaryngology and, in addition to the

Preface

full clinical cover, there are sections of physics and safety (written for the clinician) and the extremely important topic of laser safe anaesthesia. This volume should enable laser surgeons of all degrees of expertise to identify those conditions which should be treated by laser and, given the current state of knowledge, how to treat them.

J. A. S. CARRUTH FRCS
Southampton Laser Unit

1 Lasers – Physics, tissue interaction and safety

ALAN L. McKENZIE

1.1 Laser physics

1.1.1 INTRODUCTION

If lasers are ever deployed as space weapons, it will be interesting to reflect that both 'Star Wars' lasers and surgical lasers owe their efficacy not to intrinsic high power but to the phenomenon of beam parallelism. Without the ability to deliver a tight beam of radiation across hundreds of miles of space, the high-power laser weapon would be useless, while in the operating theatre, the parallelism of the surgical laser beam allows it to be focused to cut effortlessly through tissue using less power than a domestic light bulb.

It would be wrong to say altogether that the generation of high powers is not a requirement in laser surgery, because the ability of lasers to deliver all of their power at a given wavelength can be useful in instances where different tissue absorption properties can be exploited. Broadly speaking, however, in surgery, the key characteristic of laser radiation is its parallelism, enabling the beam either to be focused directly onto tissue or into a narrow optical fibre for endoscopic applications.

1.1.2 STIMULATED EMISSION

How does this beam parallelism arise? The answer is to be found in the phenomenon called stimulated emission, which Einstein predicted theoretically in 1917. Until that time, only two interaction processes were known to occur between matter and light – absorption and spontaneous emission. When a photon is absorbed by an atom, it is completely destroyed, leaving the atom in an excited state (Figure 1.1(a)). Conversely, if an atom has been given energy (by collision with an electron, for example) then it is likely that the excited atom will emit

Physics, tissue interaction and safety

this energy in the form of a photon in a random direction (Figure 1.1(b)). This is known as spontaneous emission. Einstein envisaged such an excited atom being hit by a photon of the same energy as that which normally would be emitted spontaneously. In this case the atom is stimulated to emit its energy not in a random direction, but in the very same direction as the incident photon (Figure 1.1(c)). The picture then, in stimulated emission, is of a photon interacting with an excited atom and producing as a result a copy of itself, identical in every respect. Since an atom can be excited to certain discrete energy levels only, there is a limited number of wavelengths which the stimulated photon can possess, and, by the same token, only those wavelengths can be candidates for stimulated emission.

In order to see how stimulated emission accounts for beam parallelism, imagine that a large number of excited atoms have been collected into a long, narrow cylinder with highly reflecting mirrors stuck on each of the two flat ends (Figure 1.2). When these excited atoms lose their photons by spontaneous emission, the light is generally lost out of the curved sides of the tube. Occasionally, however, a photon will be

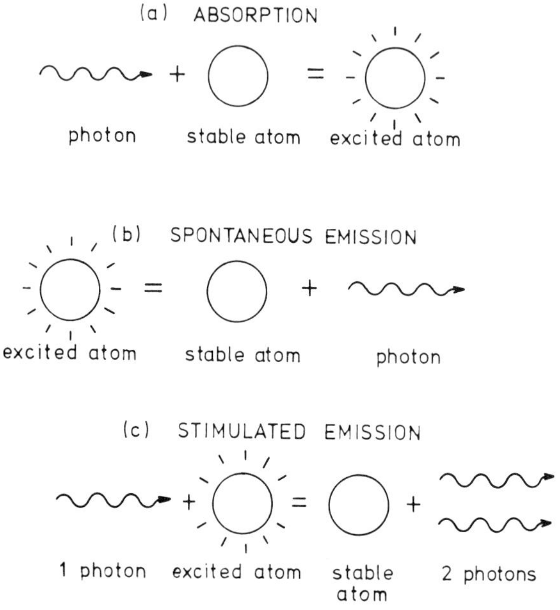

Figure 1.1 Of the three interactions, absorption, spontaneous emission and stimulated emission, the latter is the process which is responsible for laser action.

Laser physics

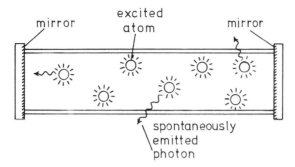

Figure 1.2 The lasing process begins when a spontaneously emitted photon is reflected along the axis of the tube, so that other photons are produced by stimulated emission.

emitted parallel to the tube axis and so it will be reflected back into the volume. Such a photon has a high chance of encountering another excited atom and stimulating it to emit another photon in the same axial direction. These two photons go on to produce another two stimulated photons, and so an avalanche builds up, with virtually all the stimulated photons travelling parallel to each other in the axial direction.

Because the original axial photon has been amplified in numbers by stimulated emission, the process gives rise to the phrase 'Light Amplification by Stimulated Emission of Radiation', from which the word 'laser' is derived as an acronym.

1.1.3 A PARALLEL BEAM OF LIGHT?

It is easy to extract a useful output beam from such a device: one of the end mirrors is simply made partially transmitting, so that some light leaks outside. This light will be emitted in a beam of about the same diameter as the volume, and all of the photons will be travelling in the same direction, which accounts for the characteristic parallelism of the laser beam.

In the nature of things, it is not possible to produce a beam which is perfectly parallel. For one thing, such a beam physically could not exist, because there would always be a tendency for it to diffract at the edges. For another, it is easier to confine the radiation within the laser tube using concave mirrors rather than flat ones, and this is frequently done in practice. But this effectively imposes a curvature upon the beam which is manifest by a divergence of the beam as it leaves the laser (Figure 1.3). A red He-Ne laser beam, used for aiming invisible surgical laser beams, could be directed straight at the moon, but the

Physics, tissue interaction and safety

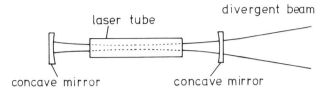

Figure 1.3 Laser beams are not absolutely parallel in practice, but diverge slightly. The degree of divergence is exaggerated here for clarity.

beam would cover a circle on the moon's surface several hundred miles across. This imperfection means that, in practice, a converging lens placed in the laser beam will not focus the radiation into an infinitely small point, but will, nevertheless, be capable of focusing a visible argon laser beam into a spot diameter of 100 μm, or a CO_2 laser beam into a circle only a millimetre or so across, depending upon the lens characteristics.

1.1.4 POPULATION INVERSION

I was once asked at a meeting of head and neck oncologists what would happen if a surgical laser beam struck a metallic instrument and was reflected directly back into the laser – would this cause the laser power inside the tube to build up without limit?

Although the conditions necessary for such an accident are unlikely, the question may be restated to ask what would happen if, instead of radiation leaking through the output mirror, suppose that both mirrors were 100% reflecting? Intuitively, of course, the radiation power inside the tube could not increase indefinitely – nature abhors infinities. But what is the actual mechanism preventing such a runaway catastrophe?

To answer this, consider the excited atoms inside the laser tube being stimulated to emit their energy in the form of laser photons. What happens to these atoms? They do not, of course, disappear, but remain in the laser tube as before. The difference is, now, that when a photon encounters the 'spent' atom, it can no longer stimulate the emission of another photon. Now the tables are turned, and the photon is liable to be absorbed by the atom, promoting it to its former excited state, called the upper laser level (Figure 1.4). If both the end mirrors were suddenly made totally reflecting, the laser power inside the tube would grow to begin with, and more excited atoms would be hit by laser photons as a consequence. This in turn, would increase the number of 'spent' atoms (called the lower laser level – Figure 1.4), and these would begin to mop up the excess laser photons by absorption. Soon an equilibrium would

Laser physics

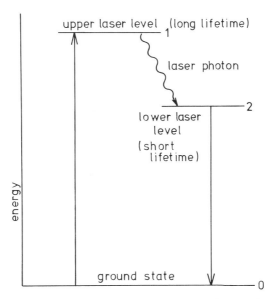

Figure 1.4 Lasing occurs when there is a greater population of atoms in a high energy state than a lower energy state. This condition is called 'population inversion'.

be reached where the numbers of upper-laser-level atoms and lower-laser-level atoms were equal, and the laser power will increase no further.

Notice that the rôle which the lower-laser-level atoms play in the production of laser light is crucial – ideally, the number of such species should be kept to a minimum, and certainly the upper-laser-level population should be greater than the lower; otherwise laser light would be absorbed as fast as it was created. This imbalance of numbers in favour of the upper laser level is called 'population inversion', because it is contrary to the normal state of affairs in a collection of excited atoms. Conditions necessary for achieving population inversion are shown in Figure 1.4. In this diagram, atoms with no excess energy are considered to be in the 'ground' state, i.e. at level 0. An atom may be excited to the upper laser level by collisions with electrons or other excited atoms in a gas discharge, or by light from outside the tube, which is termed 'optical pumping'. In order for the upper laser level (level 1) to build up, the atom in that state must have a long natural lifetime against decay by spontaneous emission or collisions with other laser atoms. By the same token, the lower laser level (level 2) will be kept small in size if the atoms there have a short lifetime against decay back

Physics, tissue interaction and safety

to the ground state. Individual laser energy-level diagrams may differ in detail from this scheme, but, in general, the broad features illustrated are common to all laser pumping schemes.

1.1.5 SPECIFIC ENT LASERS

Having discussed the general theory of laser action, let us now turn to specific examples of lasers which are used in ENT procedures. We shall consider the following lasers: CO_2; argon; Nd-YAG; dye; gold-vapour.

The output wavelengths of these lasers are shown in the spectrum in Figure 1.5. The wavelengths illustrated range from the visible, blue end of the spectrum through the near-infrared to the far-infrared. Notice that both the CO_2 and the Nd-YAG lasers are infrared-emitting devices, but that the CO_2 wavelength is exactly ten times that of the Nd-YAG.

Radiation first becomes visible in the deep red around 700 nm, and both the He-Ne and gold vapour lasers emit in the red near 630 nm. The argon beam comprises several wavelengths, especially two major ones,

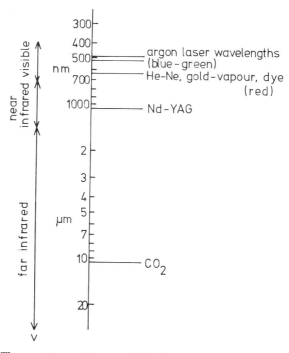

Figure 1.5 The spectrum of lasers which have been used in ENT work ranges from the blue to the far infrared.

Laser physics

at 515 nm (green) and 488 nm (blue–green). The dye laser can be tuned to give a variety of wavelengths, but, for ENT applications, as will be seen, it is set at 630 nm.

The CO_2 laser is the 'work horse' of ENT laser surgery, and, indeed, of surgery in general. It is the laser which comes nearest to substituting as a scalpel in some circumstances, although, as will be seen, to describe the CO_2 laser merely as a 'light scalpel', is to underestimate its potential. The argon laser has been used in ENT procedures to perform fine work such as stapedectomies. The Nd-YAG laser has been used to clear the upper bronchus of obstruction, and may be used generally wherever tissue needs to be cauterized or a tumour vaporized. Dye and gold-vapour lasers are in routine use in centres such as Southampton for photodynamic therapy of ENT tumours. While both lasers produce light of the correct wavelength to activate the tumourcidal drug haematoporphyrin derivative (HPD), the science and technology of all these devices are quite different, and this should be understood by the prospective user.

(a) The CO_2 laser

Principles of operation

A schematic diagram of a CO_2 laser is shown in Figure 1.6. In essence, the CO_2 laser consists simply of a discharge tube, with highly reflecting mirrors, made of germanium or silicon to reflect the far-infrared radiation. The gas inside the discharge tube is a mixture of CO_2, nitrogen and helium, although CO_2 is generally present in concentrations of less than 5%, the bulk of the mixture being helium (82%) and nitrogen (13%). These proportions are not critical, and, indeed, Hunt (1967) built

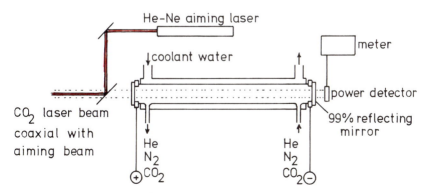

Figure 1.6 Schematic diagram of a CO_2 laser.

Physics, tissue interaction and safety

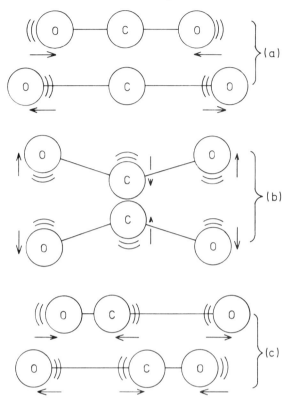

Figure 1.7 The three different modes in which a CO_2 molecule may vibrate.

a laser which ran on exhaled human breath! The principle of the CO_2 laser is exactly as we have described for the general case, only CO_2 molecules substitute for atoms in the lasing process.

The CO_2 molecule can vibrate in three independent ways (Figure 1.7). It may stretch symmetrically (Figure 1.7(a)) or bend (Figure 1.7(b)) or stretch asymmetrically (Figure 1.7(c)). Just as an atom may lose its energy by spontaneous emission, the excited CO_2 molecule can lose its vibrational energy by emitting it in the form of a photon. A molecule vibrating in the asymmetric stretch mode, however, has a relatively long lifetime, which allows the population of molecules in this state to build up. As has been seen, this is one of the necessary characteristics of an upper laser level, and this state constitutes the upper level of the 10.6 μm infrared laser transition (Figure 1.8).

This level is 'pumped' in two ways – zero energy CO_2 gas molecules collide either with fast-moving discharge electrons or with excited

Laser physics

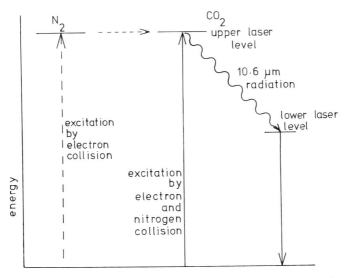

Figure 1.8 Energy level scheme for CO_2 laser operation. The upper laser level is populated both by direct discharge electron collision and by collision with excited nitrogen molecules.

nitrogen molecules. In either case, energy is transferred to the CO_2 molecules, setting them vibrating. It so happens that the vibrational energy levels of nitrogen coincide with the energy of the asymmetric stretch mode of CO_2 (Figure 1.8), which eases the transfer of energy. The nitrogen molecules, in turn, acquire their energy directly from discharge electron collisions.

The other prerequisite for lasing is that the lower laser level should have a short lifetime, so that the population of this state does not build up enough to absorb a significant amount of laser radiation. Helium, being a light, atomic gas conducts energy from the lower state and transfers it quickly to the tube walls. Effectively, the helium keeps the discharge temperature relatively low, and this prevents the build up of CO_2 molecules in the lower laser level, which would be first to suffer if the temperature rose too much.

Technology
The gas for the CO_2 laser is generally supplied ready-mixed in cylinders. These have to be replaced periodically, because the gas in the discharge tube must flow constantly to avoid the build-up of unwanted chemical species such as carbon monoxide. In order to assist the helium to cool the discharge, the tube walls are surrounded by a water jacket forming part of a closed-cycle cooling system.

Physics, tissue interaction and safety

Since the output beam is invisible, it has to be aligned with a visible beam, and, for this, a red-emitting He-Ne laser is used. The two beams are made coaxial and then are reflected by mirrors at the joints of an articulated hollow tube, designed so that the beams can emerge in any direction determined by the arm (Figure 1.9). At this stage, the surgical beam is fairly broad, and has to be focused by a lens. A zinc selenide lens is used, since this material can transmit not only the infrared surgical beam but also the visible aiming beam. The focal length of the lens depends upon the application of the surgical laser. If it is to be used in conjunction with a binocular microscope, then the lens is mounted close to the microscope objective, and will have a focal length of several hundred millimetres. If, instead, the articulated arm is terminated in a handpiece, the lens will have a shorter focal length, allowing the surgeon to work comfortably close to the operating site (Figure 1.9(a)).

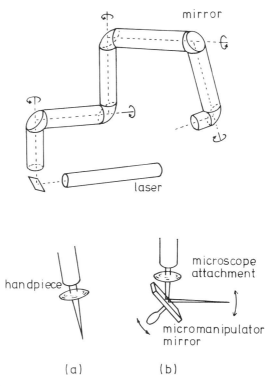

Figure 1.9 The CO_2 laser beam is directed by mirrors on the joints of an articulated tube. For surgery, the beam may be terminated either (a) in a handpiece or (b) as an attachment to a binocular microscope.

Laser physics

When the binocular microscope is used, the laser beam is directed in the operating field by a gimbal-mounted mirror and controlled by a joystick (Figure 1.9(b)). This device is called a micromanipulator, and saves the effort of having constantly to adjust the position of the binocular microscope throughout the operation. Spot sizes on the tissue surface are between 0.5 and 2 mm in diameter for a long focal length lens, and less for handpiece lenses (for a definition of spot size, see Section 1.1.6).

When the laser is operated as a scalpel (Figure 1.10(a)) the smallest spot sizes are usually the most advantageous, but if a large area of tissue is to be ablated, then the surgeon may wish to defocus the laser beam to achieve a greater tissue coverage (Figure 1.10(c)). However, as we shall see, he would then be well advised to increase the laser power accordingly, to minimize the subsurface coagulation damage. The extent of this damage is illustrated in Figures 1.10(b) and (c), and is greater where the laser power falling per unit area has been diminished by defocusing. We shall discuss the reasons for this below.

Available CO_2 laser powers vary considerably from around 20 W to 60 W or greater, depending upon the manufacturer. Originally the lasers were operated in a continuously working (CW) mode, i.e. with constant output power. However, recently, some manufacturers have introduced pulsed lasers into the market. These lasers work in bursts of

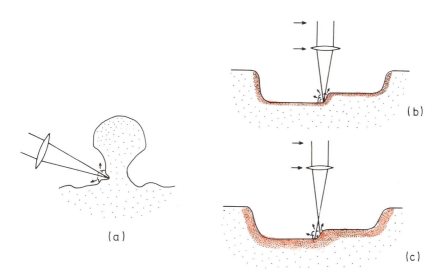

Figure 1.10 The CO_2 laser may be used either (a) to incise tissue or, (b) and (c), to ablate large areas. The extent of subsurface coagulation is indicated by the shaded area, and is greater when the laser beam is defocused.

Physics, tissue interaction and safety

several hundred to several thousand per second, and there is evidence to indicate that tissue charring may be less in such a mode. Whether the laser is CW or pulsed, the operating technique is the same – the beam may be kept on continuously while cutting or ablating, or an exposure duration may be pre-selected (for example 0.1 s, 0.2 s, 0.5 s or 1.0 s) and then the footswitch used to obtain an exposure or train of exposures.

(b) The argon laser

Principles of operation
The blue–green beam of the argon laser is emitted from argon ions rather than atoms. Ions in the upper laser level are created in two stages – an electron in the argon-gas discharge ionizes an argon atom and this ion is raised to the required energy by a second electron collision. Since the electron density in a discharge is proportional to the current going through it, and since laser level production is a two-stage process with each step depending upon an electron collision, the laser-level population is strongly current dependent, and so high currents, in the order of 30 A, are used in argon laser tubes. Population inversion is facilitated by the lower laser level having a very short natural lifetime, as ions in this level quickly decay by emitting an ultraviolet photon.

Technology
Because of the high discharge currents, the discharge tube has to be cooled by running water (Figure 1.11). Even then, the tube has to be made of materials which can withstand the heat. Previously, argon laser tubes were sometimes made of graphite, but this is vulnerable to thermal shock, and these tubes frequently broke with disastrous consequences. Modern tubes are made of ceramics which are more robust. It was found in the early days of argon lasers that a magnetic field running through the laser helped to concentrate the discharge electrons, which increased the power output. Consequently, surgical argon lasers all have solenoid windings wrapped around the central laser tube (Figure 1.11).

Because the discharge current is so high, the electrons and ions in the discharge can gather a significant momentum which results in the gas having a higher pressure at one end of the tube than the other. Since there is only one optimum pressure for any set of conditions, this tidal effect is clearly undesirable, and the problem is resolved by providing holes within the laser tube which do not carry the discharge but through which the gas can flow back to equilibrium.

The high electric fields within the argon laser discharge are capable of accelerating ions so fiercely that they can become embedded in the tube

Laser physics

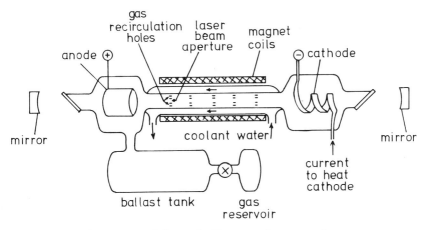

Figure 1.11 Schematic diagram of an argon laser.

walls. After many hours of use, this represents a significant loss of gas from the tube, and so a gas reservoir is usually attached to the laser tube to maintain the correct pressure. A large ballast tank (Figure 1.11) minimizes the effect of such discrete influxes of gas from time to time.

In the far-infrared there are, as yet, no very satisfactory fibres available to conduct radiation to the operating site, although a few prototypes are now in use with CO_2 lasers. However, the visible argon laser beam is transmitted with ease through an optical fibre and can be terminated either in a handpiece or in a binocular microscope. A laser fibre is not a bundle as used for imaging in an endoscope, but a single fibre of diameter 100 μm or more, and generally embedded within a strong, flexible, protective sheath. At such diameters, there is no problem in focusing the parallel beam into the end of the fibre, and when the light emerges at the other end, it is collected by a second lens which is either part of the handpiece or attached to the microscope. This lens then forms an image of the end of the fibre optic, and spot sizes as small as 50 μm may be achieved on the tissue surface.

Output powers from most surgical argon lasers are in the 3 W–5 W range, and the beam is usually delivered in exposures of 0.1–1.0 s, preselected and controlled by a footswitch-operated shutter.

(c)   The Nd-YAG laser

Principles of operation
The Nd-YAG laser is the most powerful of the surgical lasers, giving a CW output of up to 100 W. Unlike the CO_2 and the argon lasers, the

Physics, tissue interaction and safety

working medium of the Nd-YAG laser is a crystal. The crystal is yttrium aluminium garnet (YAG) and embedded in the lattice are dopant neodymium ions. The laser transition derives from excited states of the Nd ion, and the energy is provided by a powerful light source focused into the crystal rod. The lower laser level is short-lived because of interactions with the solid crystal lattice. One of the reasons for the high power capability of the Nd-YAG laser is that, being a solid, many more of the active species (Nd ions) can be packed into a given volume than if the medium were a gas.

Technology

A Nd-YAG crystal is a cylindrical rod, about 100 mm long and 6 mm in diameter. The ends of the rod are specially coated to reduce reflection losses. The light source which provides the excitation energy is typically a high-power krypton arc lamp, which has an output spectrum well matched to the absorption bands of neodymium. In order to couple light more efficiently into the crystal rod, the rod and the arc lamp are usually placed parallel and close together, with an elliptical mirror wrapped around the two, one in each focus of the ellipse (Figure 1.12).

Although the wavelength of the Nd-YAG laser beam is in the infrared, it is of a sufficiently short wavelength to be easily transmitted through an optical fibre, the universal mode of delivery of Nd-YAG laser radiation. Nd-YAG laser radiation is frequently delivered endoscopically, for example into the bronchus, by means of a fibre inserted through the biopsy channel.

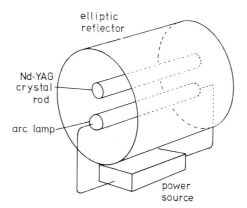

Figure 1.12 Schematic diagram of a Nd-YAG laser.

Laser physics

(d) The dye laser

Principles of operation

The dye laser is used in ENT photodynamic procedures to produce red light which excites tumourcidal HPD. The principal feature of the dye laser is that it can be tuned to lase at any wavelength in the visible, near-ultraviolet or near-infrared. This facility arises because the dye is an organic molecule comprising many atoms, so that the molecule can have many independent modes of vibration. This variety gives rise to a spectrum of potential laser lines, and any given dye is able to lase over a range of wavelengths spanning some 50 nm, so that the laser wavelength requirements dictate the choice of dye. Fine tuning within the 50 nm band is accomplished by inserting a tuning element between the laser mirrors. This could be a prism, but, in some designs, a special crystal known as a birefringent crystal is used, which allows only one wavelength of light to pass through it depending upon the angle at which it is fitted (Figure 1.13).

Technology

The energy to excite the dye molecules is provided by an external light source. The dye is highly absorbing, and a configuration such as is used for the Nd-YAG laser would not be practicable. Only by focusing a laser beam into a tiny spot in the dye can the necessary level of intensity be achieved, and so an argon laser is used to pump the dye laser in photodynamic therapy.

In order to avoid temperature effects, the dye must be circulated. It can either be directed through a narrow cell where the argon beam can be focused onto it, or it can be squirted through a nozzle forming a fine jet which is then caught, and the dye is returned to the reservoir. This

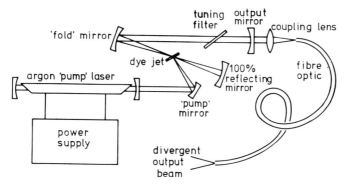

Figure 1.13 Schematic diagram of an argon pumped dye laser.

Physics, tissue interaction and safety

jet can then be illuminated by the pumping laser beam, the advantage of the jet being that reflecting, loss making surfaces of the dye-cell walls are eliminated.

As a rule of thumb, dye lasers convert between 20 and 25% of the pumping laser power into laser light of the selected wavelength. A common configuration is for a 5 W argon laser to pump a dye laser to produce about 1 W of output laser radiation, and correspondingly greater powers may be derived from an arrangement of two argon lasers focused simultaneously onto the dye jet.

The laser output is delivered to the treatment site via an optical fibre. Since the aim of photodynamic therapy is not to raise the temperature of the tumour so much as to deliver radiation uniformly to the volume, there is no need to focus the output from the fibre. The light diverges from the fibre with a cone angle of between 10° and 15°, and it is usually adequate simply to suspend the fibre sufficiently far from the tissue surface that the whole treatment site is bathed in red light. Appropriate measures can be taken to ensure uniformity of illumination using this technique (McKenzie, 1984). Alternatively, the fibre can be inserted directly into the tumour mass, and the light will then diffuse from the fibre and irradiate the tumour from within. There are ways of relating the dose delivered in this fashion to that delivered by an external fibre (McKenzie, 1985).

Users of dye lasers have expressed frustration at the difficulties of achieving a stable power output – by their nature, dye lasers are optically more complicated than other clinical lasers. The chief problems centre around keeping the argon pump laser aligned on the correct area of the dye jet, the adjustment of the dye laser mirrors, and the many surfaces in the dye laser which can become dirty and result in lost power. These problems are not insuperable, but, at present, it would be wise for a clinician embarking upon photoradiation therapy using a dye laser to ensure that technical support is readily available.

(e) The gold-vapour laser

Principles of operation
The other laser capable of exciting HPD at a respectable power (1 W or greater) is the gold-vapour laser, although this cannot be tuned and its output remains fixed at 628 nm. The gold-vapour laser is so called because the laser transition derives from gold atoms which are present as a vapour at high temperature in the discharge tube. The discharge is carried by a gas such as helium or, more usually, neon, and the discharge tube is heavily insulated (Figure 1.14) so that the temperature eventually becomes great enough to vaporize snippets of gold wire laid along the tube at intervals.

Laser physics

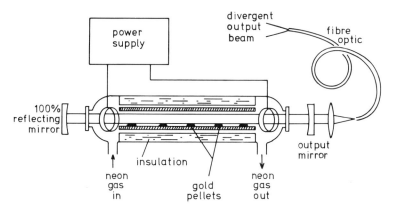

Figure 1.14 Schematic diagram of a gold-vapour laser.

The characteristic feature of the gold-vapour laser is that it is pulsed, although these pulses are so rapid (about 10 kHz) that, to all intents and purposes, the beam is effectively continuous. The reason for pulsing is that the lower laser level breaks one of the prime laser rules – it has a long lifetime. Only when the discharge first switches on does the upper laser level predominate in numbers: the lower laser level builds up as fast as the upper level decays, and lasing can only take place for a few tens of nanoseconds after the discharge is turned on. The only way out is to close down the discharge, allowing the gold atoms to lose their energy, and to go through the cycle again – many thousands of times per second.

Technology
Pulsing is not a disadvantage in photodynamic therapy, because the biological effect is cumulative, and does not depend upon peak power. The only consequence is that the power supply has to be slightly more sophisticated in order to switch the high voltages at the required frequency. Unlike the dye laser, the optics of the gold-vapour laser are very simple and require virtually no attention. The gold in the laser tends to become redistributed after many hours of use, and should either be reclaimed and reinserted, or new wire should be used in its place. This latter procedure is not a particularly expensive philosophy because the amount of gold 'lost' per patient is in practice small.

A remarkable feature of the gold-vapour laser is its beam diameter, which can be very wide, usually 25 mm or more. However, this can be focused into a narrow optical fibre and used in the same way as described for the dye laser. Gold-vapour lasers can be 'portable' in as much as they are available in models which need no water cooling and

Physics, tissue interaction and safety

can be plugged into a domestic electricity socket. Such a device will give an average output of about 1.5 W. There are powerful versions which give up to 9 W, but these need water mains and three-phase electricity connections. An insurance policy with these lasers is that, should a better substance than HPD be developed, requiring excitation at a different wavelength, the laser can easily be converted to running on copper, lasing at 510 nm and 578 nm, which can then drive a dye laser tuned to the new wavelength. Copper produces a more powerful beam than the gold system, so that the dye laser output power will be comparable with that obtained with gold, and still well in excess of that generally found with argon-pumped dye lasers.

1.1.6 SPOT SIZES AND IRRADIANCE

For all medical and surgical applications, it is important to know not simply the power or energy applied to tissue, but also the power per unit area of tissue irradiated. Evidently, a given power delivered to a small area of tissue will be more effective within the boundaries of the laser spot than the same power spread over a larger area. The quantity which incorporates both power and area is the 'irradiance' which expresses the power delivered per unit area in W/m^2 or W/mm^2. (Irradiance is also known, popularly, as 'power density'.)

The area irradiated by the laser beam is defined by the 'spot size', which requires some explanation. Seen in cross section, a laser beam is normally circular, although some manufacturers of CO_2 lasers offer beams which have a more complicated structure such as a circle split down the middle, or even a circle with a hole in the middle. The patterns are called modes, and the most common, circular mode is called the TEM_{00} mode.

If the laser radiation is collected and focused directly by a lens, as in the CO_2 laser (as opposed to the argon laser where it is the light diverging from an optical fibre which is focused), the circle of radiation is reduced to a minimum size at the focal point. The diameter of this circle is termed the spot diameter, or spot size. Since the TEM_{00} mode does not exhibit a sharp cutoff, the diameter is measured beween the points where the power has fallen to 14% of its central value, for reasons of optical physics. This mathematical convenience does not prevent the laser radiation having some effect beyond the notional boundary, and so the diameters of charred craters in soft tissue or in a wooden spatula may well be larger than the quoted spot size. However, the spot size gives a working guide to the extent of the irradiated area, and the concept may also be usefully applied to other laser mode patterns and to the case of optical fibre delivery.

Laser–tissue interaction

Other things being equal, spot sizes are smallest with lenses of short focal length. Thus a typical spot for a CO_2 laser handpiece, incorporating a 75 mm lens, may be 150 μm in diameter, whereas a 400 mm lens used in conjunction with an operating microscope will produce a spot size of 0.5–1.5 mm.

The irradiance for any exposure is averaged over the laser spot by dividing the beam power by the area calculated from the spot diameter. If the laser is defocused, the spot size on the treatment site will be larger and the irradiance correspondingly less. Since the value of the irradiance generally determines the effect of the beam upon tissue, it should be quoted wherever appropriate, or at least the necessary parameters should be given so that the reader can derive it himself.

1.2 Laser–tissue interaction

1.2.1 INTRODUCTION

The interaction of laser radiation with tissue may be categorized into thermal and non-thermal processes. Examples of non-thermal processes are the photomechanical effect and the photochemical effect. The photomechanical effect is principally confined to the use of pulsed Nd-YAG ophthalmic surgery where the high irradiance of the strongly focused beam causes a miniature ball of plasma to be created momentarily at the target. The shockwaves from this plasma disrupt the target, which is generally a semitransparent membrane such as vitreous strands or an opacified posterior or anterior capsule. The photochemical effect exploits the energy of laser photons to interact directly with molecules to break tissue bonding or to activate a cytotoxic drug.

An instance of the former photochemical process is the use of UV lasers to shape the cornea or to remove atherosclerotic plaque from diseased vessels. However, the only use of a non-thermal process in laser ENT work is the photochemical activation of a drug such as HPD, by a gold laser or a dye laser tuned to 630 nm. This will be discussed in more detail in Chapter 9, and we shall now consider those processes under which all other ENT laser procedures may be categorized – the thermal effects of laser radiation on tissue.

1.2.2 THERMAL EFFECTS

When laser radiation is incident upon tissue, it is absorbed to a greater or lesser extent, and the temperature of the tissue rises. When the temperature of soft tissue rises from 37°C to about 60°C, no change in

Physics, tissue interaction and safety

the tissue structure is discernible if the temperature rise is of short duration. Above 60°C, soft tissue begins to coagulate.

(a) Coagulation

Of particular importance in the coagulation process is the behaviour of collagen. When collagen fibres reach temperatures greater than 60°C, the protein begins to denature, undergoing a structural deformation, a kind of phase transition. On a molecular level, this is due to the protein chains which constitute the collagen becoming randomized. This change is manifest by light being more readily scattered by the randomized protein chains. This accounts for the appearance of egg 'white' and the blanching of steak or liver as it is fried.

Concomitant with the randomization is a shrinkage of the collagen chains. This may be observed macroscopically in the wrinkling of bacon as it is grilled. Collagen shrinkage accounts for the haemostatic property of a laser beam – as the perivascular collagenous sheaths of blood vessels increase in temperature, they shrink, and the blood supply is reduced or cut off. Gorisch and Boergen (1982) showed that, under tension due to pressure from the circulating blood, the temperature at which shrinkage begins is above 70°C for veins and 75°C for arteries. In practice, shrinkage of the connective tissue in which the vessels are embedded will contribute to the haemostasis, and clotting due to thrombocytic action on heat-damaged erythrocytes may be considered a secondary cause, although not a primary one.

(b) Vaporization

When the temperature of soft tissue is raised to 100°C the water in cells can boil. The conversion of water into steam represents an expansion of a thousandfold, and since, for a given cell at normal surgical laser powers, this is virtually instantaneous, the cell walls are disrupted explosively. Tissue which has been ablated in this way is commonly said to have been 'vaporized'.

(c) Burning

Once the water has been removed from the irradiated cells, any debris remaining will quickly rise in temperature, blackening and outgassing in the process. At around 400°C–500°C this residual material will be burnt, but since it will not be in good thermal contact with the bulk of the tissue, this does not represent a source of damage for the underlying healthy tissue.

Laser–tissue interaction

The reaction of soft tissue to heat as considered in the general manner presented above will form the background to a more detailed examination of laser–tissue interaction with regard to individual laser types.

1.2.3 CO_2 LASER RADIATION

The characteristic feature of CO_2 laser radiation is that the far-infrared, 10.6 μm beam is absorbed very strongly by water, and, hence, soft tissue. The figure normally used is that of Kiefhaber, Nath and Moritz (1977) who give an absorption coefficient of 200/cm. This means that a CO_2 laser beam will be 90% absorbed in a distance of only 100 μm or so. In consequence the laser energy is confined to a small volume, and the local temperature quickly rises to boiling point, vaporizing this top 100 μm layer of cells. This exposes the subjacent tissue which is vaporized in like fashion. As each successive layer of tissue is vaporized and removed by the laser beam, so the next is exposed and vaporized in its turn. The important point about this process is that the temperature of the irradiated surface never exceeds 100°C, which limits the spread of thermal damage beneath the surface. Once the tissue has reached boiling point, all the extra input of laser power goes to converting water into steam – the power is used to provide 'latent' heat of vaporization rather than to raise the temperature beyond 100°C.

Deep craters and incisions are produced not by the penetration of radiation directly into the tissue, but by the successive vaporization of exposed layers. The speed with which a crater may be 'drilled' depends upon the irradiance (power per unit area) of the laser beam. A 10 W beam focused into a spot of area 1 mm^2 will, according to Litwin *et al.* (1969) produce a crater 1 mm deep in 0.1 s.

(a) Subsurface damage

Although the CO_2 laser beam penetrates only about 100 μm into soft tissue, the heat which is concentrated at the incised surface will tend to spread by conduction more deeply into the bulk of the tissue, and the extent of this can be seen from the depth of coagulation beneath the surface of the excision. Calculations show (McKenzie, 1983) that, at typical values of beam concentration and pulse duration, tissue is coagulated by heat diffusion to a depth of several hundred micrometres – and even up to one millimetre – below the surface (Figure 1.15). This has implications, of course, for the haemostatic efficiency of the laser excision process, as well as for the efficacy of post-operative healing. In general, the higher the concentration of power in the laser spot, the less will be the depth of coagulation, because, broadly speaking, the extra

Physics, tissue interaction and safety

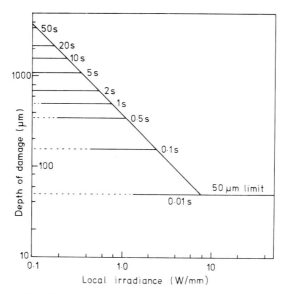

Figure 1.15 Graph showing the depth of coagulation beneath a CO_2 laser incision. This is indicated by the position on the diagonal line corresponding to a given irradiance. The depth of damage may be limited by the time available for heat to diffuse, found from the horizontal line appropriate to the indicated exposure duration.

energy is used more efficiently in vaporizing rather than being conducted away to coagulate. In practical terms, it is inadvisable to defocus the beam in order to cover larger areas more quickly, without increasing the beam power accordingly; otherwise the depth of coagulation will be increased by defocusing.

1.2.4 Nd-YAG LASER RADIATION

In one respect Nd-YAG and CO_2 laser radiation are at opposite extremes of the interaction scale. In contrast to the local absorption property of the CO_2 laser beam, the Nd-YAG beam is relatively poorly absorbed, and, instead, is scattered and diffused by tissue inhomogeneities. So great is the scattering/absorption ratio that, in soft tissue, the YAG beam is almost completely diffuse in character. A photon of the near-infrared radiation may be scattered many times before finally being absorbed, and so a beam which enters the tissue surface at a given point can heat tissue directly several millimetres away (Figure 1.16).

Because the effect of the Nd-YAG laser beam is diffuse, affecting a large volume of tissue in comparison with the amount affected by a CO_2

Laser–tissue interaction

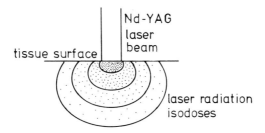

Figure 1.16 A Nd-YAG laser beam diffuses several millimetres from its point of entry in soft tissue.

laser beam, the temperature rise for a similar energy input is far less in the case of the Nd-YAG laser. Nd-YAG lasers tend, as a consequence, to be run at higher powers (60 W–100 W) than the CO_2 laser (20 W–60 W), but, even so, the instant vaporization characteristics of the CO_2 beam are not found in the case of the Nd-YAG beam. Instead, the tissue heats up more slowly, and the desired result is frequently, although not always, coagulation of a bleeding ulcer or tumour, rather than vaporization. If the Nd-YAG beam is applied for long enough, boiling point will be reached, and tissue vaporized in this way will have, surrounding it, a capsule of coagulation far greater in thickness than would be found beneath a CO_2 laser incision.

1.2.5 ARGON LASER RADIATION

The blue–green beam of the argon laser is scattered even more than that of the Nd-YAG laser beam. However, the effect of absorption by some 'chromophores' such as blood also becomes more significant, so that the overall penetration of the argon beam in soft tissue is less than that of the Nd-YAG laser beam. A smaller volume of tissue is affected, therefore, by an argon beam than by a Nd-YAG beam. Since the energy is distributed in a smaller volume, it clearly requires less energy to induce coagulation with an argon laser than with a Nd-YAG. On the other hand, the smaller penetration depth means that, whereas the Nd-YAG laser can seal vessels of up to 1.5 mm in diameter, the argon laser is only successful for vessels of up to 1 mm (Kelly et al., 1983).

The selective absorption of the argon laser beam by blood can be exploited in cases where vascular tissue is to be coagulated, sparing the surrounding avascular tissue. Hence, for example, cutaneous haemangiomas can be treated through overlying, non-coloured cutaneous structures, and coagulation of minute blood vessels lying in nerve fibres (vasonervorum) or on the surface of vital structures becomes a possibil-

Physics, tissue interaction and safety

ity (di Bartolomeo, 1981). Essentially, the blue–green beam is strongly absorbed by the red blood, whereas it tends to diffuse harmlessly away in the non-coloured tissues. More energy is therefore deposited in vascularized tissue which experiences a greater temperature rise than the avascular tissue. The skill is in delivering sufficient energy to coagulate the blood-bearing structures without giving such a high dose that the whole field is obliterated, regardless of constitution.

1.3 Laser safety

INTRODUCTION

A surgical laser is dangerous for two reasons: it can destroy human tissue directly and it can ignite combustible materials. Laser safety philosophy evaluates means of minimizing these hazards, in particular, how to protect the eye from exposure to the laser beam and how to administer anaesthetic gases in comparative safety in the presence of laser radiation. The considerations relating to the latter problem are extensive, and detailed discussion is given in Chapter 2.

Accidental exposure to laser radiation in an operating theatre may occur in two ways: either directly from the laser itself or by reflection from tissue or instruments. A likely example of the former event is for the surgeon to irradiate his own hand or that of a colleague while it is within the operating field, or, alternatively, to step inadvertently on the footswitch while adjusting the laser which is aimed momentarily at an unfortunate member of the theatre staff.

1.3.2 REFLECTIONS

In considering exposure by reflection, we must distinguish between specular, mirror-like reflection and diffuse reflection. Specular reflection arises from smooth surfaces, in particular from metallic instruments. Like visible light, the infrared beam of the CO_2 laser is highly reflected by metallic surfaces. Instruments are available with roughened, matt surfaces but it should be remembered that a surface which appears matt in visible light is not necessarily so at CO_2 laser wavelengths, and due caution should be exercised in the use of instruments surfaced in this way.

Diffusely reflected radiation results from a beam striking a rough surface, which scatters the energy in all directions. Most surfaces are diffusely reflecting, such as human tissue (although a film of blood can specularly reflect the red beam of a dye or gold-vapour laser), swabs and

Laser safety

towels, and theatre walls (although these can be specularly reflecting when gloss painted).

Essentially, the result of human tissue exposure to laser radiation is a burn if the irradiance ('power density') is great enough. Because of the large, exposed surface, there is a greater probability that a misdirected beam will hit the skin of a member of the theatre staff than the eye. However, a skin burn produced in this way is a minor irritation compared with the potentially disastrous repercussions of an eye exposure. Consequently, while due care must be taken by the surgeon to avoid directing the beam or its specular reflection in the vicinity of other personnel, more positive action is required to protect the eyes.

1.3.3 EFFECT OF LASER RADIATION ON THE EYE

The effect of laser radiation upon the eye depends upon the laser wavelength. The far-infrared CO_2 laser beam is completely absorbed within a 100 μm or so of soft tissue, so that transitory exposure to the beam will only result in a corneal burn, at worst (see Figure 1.17). If it is fairly superficial, the white, opaque scar should disappear within a day or so, once the corneal epithelial cells have regenerated. The near-infrared YAG beam and the visible beams of argon, dye and gold-vapour lasers will all be transmitted through the ocular media to the retina where, if the irradiance is great enough, permanent damage will elicit a scotoma in the victim's field of vision.

Exposure to laser radiation is divided into two categories termed 'intrabeam' and 'extended-source'. An intrabeam exposure occurs in the direct or specularly reflected laser beam, whereas extended-source exposure refers to exposure from diffusely reflected radiation from a

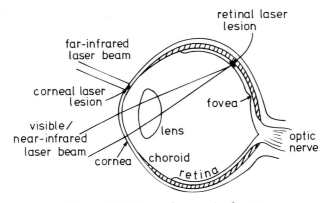

Figure 1.17 Laser damage in the eye.

Physics, tissue interaction and safety

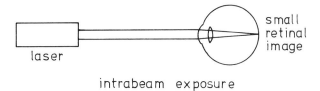

intrabeam exposure

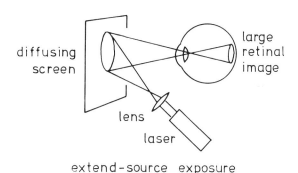

extend-source exposure

Figure 1.18 Illustrating the difference between intrabeam and extended-source exposure.

comparatively wide area. The two concepts are illustrated in Figure 1.18.

1.3.4 MAXIMUM PERMISSIBLE EXPOSURE

Much experimental work has been done to determine the risk thresholds for different wavelengths and exposure durations, and there is broad international agreement over the values of these thresholds in terms of beam irradiance at the eye. The data have been summarized in the form of tables of Maximum Permissible Exposure (MPE) for both intrabeam and extended-source conditions. In practice, it is only necessary to take account of the intrabeam tables, which refer to the concentrated radiation beam, since an eye which is protected according to these tables will certainly be safe from diffuse reflection. An example from the MPE tables is shown in Table 1.1.

MPE data have been used to classify lasers according to the danger they present, ranging from the innocuous Class I lasers to the extremely hazardous Class IV devices, which have powers of greater than 0.5 W. All ENT surgical lasers are Class IV devices, apart from the red He-Ne laser aiming beam incorporated into CO_2 and Nd-YAG lasers. These

Laser safety

Table 1.1 Maximum permissible exposure for three wavelength ranges commonly used in surgery

Wavelength (nm)	Maximum permissible corneal exposure (J/m²)
400–700 (visible)	$18\ t^{0.75}$
1050–1400 (near infrared)	$90\ t^{0.75}$
1400–10⁶ (far infrared)	$5600\ t^{0.25}$

Valid for exposure durations, t, between 50×10^{-6} s and 10 s.

aiming lasers are in the Class II category, which means that a momentary eye exposure is safe, but, of course, they must not be stared into. The classification is summarized in Table 1.2.

1.3.5 EYE PROTECTION

In order to obviate the possibility of eye exposure to levels greater than the MPE, properly designed eye protection must be worn. This must conform with two criteria:

1. The filters in the eyewear must attenuate the laser beam sufficiently that even direct exposure to the beam will not exceed the MPE at the eye.
2. The filters must be designed to withstand the highest values of irradiance available from the laser without puncturing or shattering.

Table 1.2 Classification of CW lasers

Class I	Powers not to exceed MPE for eye
Class II	Visible laser beams only. Powers up to 1 mW. Eye protected by blink reflex time of 0.25 s.
Class IIIa	Relaxation of Class II to 5 mW for visible radiation provided beam is expanded so that eye is still protected by blink reflex.
IIIb	Powers up to 0.5 W. Direct viewing hazardous.
Class IV	Powers over 0.5 W. Extremely hazardous.

Physics, tissue interaction and safety

The first criterion is easily met, and various national regulations demand that suitable eyewear be inscribed with the degree of attenuation and the wavelength for which protection is afforded. More difficult to fulfil, however, is the second requirement, and few manufacturers will provide such certification of their product. Nevertheless, appropriate eyewear, properly documented, is available, and should be procured wherever possible.

If the surgeon is using a binocular microscope to operate with a CO_2 laser, then he need not wear eye protection, as the glass optics of the microscope will absorb any reflection directed back towards the instrument. All other personnel must wear eye protection at CO_2 laser procedures, and the patient's eyes should be protected by, for example, moist swabs taped over the closed lids. If the CO_2 laser radiation is delivered via a handpiece, then the surgeon should also wear eye protection.

In argon laser operations, all attendant staff must again use the appropriate eyewear. If the argon laser is coupled to a binocular microscope, then that microscope must have fitted to it, by the laser supplier, filters which are activated during laser exposure to prevent reflected light being transmitted back to the surgeon's eyes.

Nd-YAG laser procedures are generally performed using an optical fibre introduced into a bronchoscope. There will normally be a filter on the eyepiece of the endoscope to protect the viewer against retroreflected Nd-YAG radiation – this, of course must not be removed during an operation. Since the fibre is frequently withdrawn to clear the tip of debris, and since it may slip out of the endoscope during the procedure, the patient and attendant staff should wear eye protection.

Laser photodynamic therapy is delivered via an optical fibre held either above or implanted into the tumour to be treated. For laser powers around 1 W it may be considered reasonable to waive the wearing of goggles. A chance exposure to the divergent beam which emerges from the end of the optical fibre will not necessarily exceed the MPE for the eye (McKenzie and Carruth, 1984), and the disadvantage of wearing eye protection is that the blue filters make it impossible to see where the red beam is being aimed on the patient's tissue. Prudence dictates, however, that the patient himself, since he is not normally anaesthetized for these procedures, should wear eye protection.

1.3.6 ORGANIZATION

The procurement of the correct eyewear, and the organization of laser safety in general, should be delegated to a physicist with some experience in these matters. It is the duty of the employing authority to ensure

Laser safety

that a satisfactory mechanism is established to oversee the safety of all the lasers within its jurisdiction. In the UK, the Department of Health and Social Security has recommended (DHSS, 1984) the appointment of a Laser Protection Adviser (LPA). He should sit on the Radiation Safety Committee, which is normally concerned with X-radiation safety, and would be responsible for laser safety policy within his region or district. He should see that safety codes are written for all new and existing lasers within his control, and that these codes are observed whenever the lasers are used. For each laser or laser theatre he should appoint a Laser Protection Supervisor (LPS) who will be able to attend the laser sessions regularly, and who could be, for example, a theatre sister or staff nurse, or even the surgeon himself.

The Laser Protection Supervisor will collaborate with the Laser Protection Adviser in devising the safety code – he will often have a better appreciation of local circumstances and problems than the LPA, and his input is invaluable. When a laser is to be used in theatre, the LPS will make the correct eyewear available, and see that all personnel are provided with a pair. It is particularly important that eyewear of the correct type is identified and selected where there is more than one type of laser on site, e.g. a CO_2 laser and an argon laser, since the infrared filters of CO_2 laser goggles are transparent to blue–green argon laser radiation. The LPS will check that suitable warning signs or lights are in position outside the laser theatre door, and that a pan of water or saline is available in case of fire. He should ensure that moist swabs are taped in place over the anaesthetized patient's eyes, or that conscious patients are given the appropriate goggles to wear. Any safety problems which arise should be referred to the LPS in the first instance, and, if he cannot deal with them, he will, in turn, transmit them to the LPA.

1.3.7 SAFETY CODES

The safety code drawn up by the LPA in collaboration with the LPS is a set of rules and information containing a mixture of general advice and requirements specific to a particular laser or laser theatre. The code will usually be divided into three sections.

1. General description of the hazards
2. Administrative procedures
3. Practical safety procedures

(a) General description of the hazards

This section will describe the laser to be used (e.g. 'a 40 W CO_2 laser emitting an invisible infrared beam aligned with a 0.8 mW red He–Ne

Physics, tissue interaction and safety

laser beam') and the danger (e.g. 'burns to the skin and the cornea of the eye can result from exposure to the CO_2 laser beam or its reflection').

(b) Administrative procedures

This part of the code will list the agreed nominated users of the machine. In addition to surgeons, this may also include a theatre nurse if it is policy for such an assistant to operate the power and time settings. Service engineers will also require access.

Information should also be given on where to obtain the key to the system. This may be held by a theatre sister, or the Laser Protection Supervisor, or perhaps one of the surgeons.

The concept of Laser Controlled Area should be introduced at this stage. The Laser Controlled Area is the area – normally the operating theatre – where the safety code applies, but, since the area may not always be used for laser procedures, a more careful definition should be made. It is usually satisfactory to define the Laser Controlled Area as the room in which the laser is to be used whenever the mains power to the laser is on.

(c) Practical safety procedures

This section contains the 'meat' of the safety code. It is here that the requirement for all theatre staff to wear the correct eye protection will be stipulated. The surgeon will be exempted if he is working through a binocular microscope (fitted with the appropriate filters in the case of argon laser surgery). The responsibility of the surgeon will be made clear – ultimately, the safety of the patient and the theatre staff are in his hands. Advice will be given, such as not switching on the laser until it is approximately aimed within the operating field. This should be kept clear of unnecessary reflecting instruments. The surgeon should warn theatre staff when he is about to begin the laser procedures. Whenever there is a natural break in treatment, the rules should require that the laser be temporarily disabled by switching to 'stand by' mode if this is possible.

Finally, the safety code should require that the LPA be informed in the event of an incident as soon as possible, and a contact telephone number should be given. Examples of local rules may be found in Carruth, McKenzie and Wainwright (1980), Stamp (1983) and Davison (1983).

1.3.8 CONCLUSION

Laser safety in hospitals has enjoyed a relatively clean record. However, with the increasing efficacy of laser operations, the proliferation of

Further reading

lasers in recent years and the involvement of many more staff at laser procedures, the potential for a laser accident has risen enormously. Provided, nevertheless, that laser safety is organized and understood along lines such as those sketched above, the outlook for a trouble-free future in laser surgery remains bright.

References

Carruth, J. A. S., McKenzie, A. L. and Wainwright, A. C. (1980), The carbon dioxide laser: safety aspects. *J. Laryngol. Otol.*, **94**, 411–17.

Davison, M. (1983), Local rules for treatment lasers. *Proc. 1st Annual Conference of the British Medical Laser Association*. London.

Department of Health and Social Security (1984), *Guidance on the safe use of lasers in medical practice*. HMSO, London.

di Bartolomeo, J. R. (1981), The argon and CO_2 lasers in otolaryngology: which one and why? *Laryngoscope*, Suppl. 26, **41**, 1–16.

Gorisch, W. and Boergen, K. P. (1982) Heat induced contraction of blood vessels. *Lasers Surg. Med.*, **2**, 1–13.

Hunt, D. J. (1967), Laser action in human breath and its use for monitoring the carbon dioxide content of the air. *J. Sci. Instr.*, **44**, 408–10.

Kelly, D. F., Bown, S. G., Calder, B. M., Pearson, H., Weaver, B. M. Q., Swain, C. P. and Salmon, P. R. (1983), Historical changes following Nd-YAG laser photocoagulation of canine gastric mucosa. *Gut*, **24**, 914–20.

Kiefhaber, P., Nath, G. and Moritz, K. (1972), Endoscopical control of massive gastrointestinal haemorrhage by irradiation with a high-power Neodymium YAG laser. *Progr. Surg.*, **15**, 140–55.

Litwin, M. S., Fine, S., Klein, E. and Fine, B. S. (1969), Burn injury after carbon dioxide laser irradiation. *Arch. Surg.*, **98**, 219–22.

McKenzie, A. L. (1983), How far does thermal damage extend beneath the surface of CO_2 laser incisions? *Phys. Med. Biol.*, **28**, 905–12.

McKenzie, A. L. (1984), How to control beam profile during laser photoradiation therapy. *Phys. Med. Biol.*, **29**, 53–6.

McKenzie, A. L. (1985), How may external and interstitial illumination be compared in laser photodynamic therapy? *Phys. Med. Biol.*, **30**, 455–60.

McKenzie, A. L. and Carruth, J. A. S. (1984), Lasers in surgery and medicine. *Phys. Med. Biol.*, **29**, 619–41.

Stamp, J. M. (1983), An introduction to medical lasers. *Clin. Phys. Physiol. Measurement*, **1**, 267–90.

Further reading

PHYSICS AND TECHNOLOGY

Beach, A. D. (1969), A laser manipulator for surgical use. *J. Sci. Inst.*, sec. 2, **2**, 931–2.

Bloom, A. L. (1968), *Gas Lasers*. John Wiley and Sons, Chichester.

Bridges, W. B. (1964), Laser oscillation in singly ionised argon in the visible

spectrum. *Appl. Phys. Lett.*, **4**, 128–30.
Geusic, J. E., Marcos, H. M. and Van Uitert, L. G. (1964), Laser oscillations in Nd-doped yttrium aluminium, yttrium gallium and yttrium gadolinium garnets. *Appl. Phys. Lett.*, **4**, 182–4.
Goodwin, D. W. and Heavens, O. S. (1968), Doped crystal and gas lasers *Rep. Progr. Phys.*, **31**, 777–859.
Kamiryo, K., Kano, T. and Hidenori, K. (1966), Optimum design of elliptical pumping chambers for solid lasers. *Jpn. J. Appl. Phys.*, **5**, 1217–26.
Maitland, A. and Dunn, M. H. (1969), *Laser Physics*. North-Holland, Amsterdam.
Paananen, R. A. (1966), Progress in ionised argon lasers. *IEEE Spectrum*, **3**, 88–99.
Patel, C. K. N. (1964), Continuous-wave laser action on vibrational-rotational transitions of CO_2. *Phys. Rev.*, **136A**, 1187–93.
Peterson, O. G., Tuccio, S. A. and Snavely, B. B. (1970), CW operation of an organic dye solution laser. *Appl. Phys. Lett.*, **17**, 245–7.
Shank, C. V. (1975), Physics of dye lasers. *Rev. Modern Phys.*, **47**, 649–57.

LASER–TISSUE INTERACTION

Aronoff, B. L. (1978), CO_2 laser in surgical oncology. *Int. Adv. Surg. Oncol.*, **1**, 243–63.
Bellina, J. H. and Seto, Y. J. (1980), Pathological and physical investigations into CO_2 laser-tissue interactions with specific emphasis on cervical intraepithelial neoplasm. *Lasers Surg. Med.*, **1**, 47–69.
Dougherty, T. J., Kaufman, J. E., Goldfarb, A., Weishaupt, K. R., Boyle, D. and Mittleman, A. (1978), Photoradiation therapy for the treatment of malignant tumours. *Cancer Res.*, **38**, 2628–35.
Haldorsson, T. and Langerholc, J. (1978), Thermodynamic analysis of laser irradiation of biological tissue. *Appl. Optics*, **17**, 3943–58.
Hall, R. R., Beach, A. D., Baker, E. and Morison, P. C. A. (1971) Incision of tissue by carbon dioxide laser. *Nature*, **232**, 131–2.
Kroy, W., Haldorsson, T. and Langerholc, J. (1980), Laser coagulation: practical advice from a theoretical viewpoint. *Appl. Optics*, **19**, 6–9.
McKenzie, A. L. (1986), A three-zone model of soft-tissue damage by a CO_2 laser. *Phys. Med. Biol.*, **31**, 967–83.
Mihashi, S., Jako, G., Incze, J., Strong, M. S. and Vaughan, C. W. (1976), Laser surgery in otolaryngology: interaction of CO_2 laser and soft tissue. *Ann. NY Acad. Sci.*, **267**, 263–95.
Profio, A. E. and Doiron, D. R. (1981), Dosimetry considerations in phototherapy. *Med. Phys.*, **8**, 190–6.
Svaasand, L. O., Doiron, D. R. and Profio, A. E. (1981), *Light Distribution in Tissue during Photoradiation Therapy*. Medical Imaging Science Group, University of Southern California. USC–MISG 900–02 April.
Verschueren, R. (1976), *The CO_2 Laser in Tumour Surgery*. Van Gorcum.

Further reading

SAFETY

American National Standards Institute (1976), *Safe Use of Lasers*. Standard Z-136. New York.

British Standards Institution (1983), *Radiation Safety of Laser Products and Systems* BS 4803 parts 1-3. HMSO, London.

Decker, C. D. (1977), Accident victim's view. *Laser Focus*, **13** (8), 6.

Ham, W. T., Mueller, H. A. and Sliney, D. H. (1976), Retinal sensitivity to damage from short-wavelength light. *Nature*, **260**, 153-4.

Hayes, J. R. and Wolbarsht, M. L. (1968), Thermal model for retinal damage induced by pulsed lasers. *Aerospace Med.*, **39** (5), 474.

Sliney, D. H. (1980), Laser safety: past and present problem areas in *Lasers in Biology and Medicine* (ed. F. Hillenkamp, R. Pratesi and C. A. Sacchi) Plenum Press, New York.

Sliney, D. H. and Wolbarsht, M. L. (1980), *Safety with Lasers and Other Optical Sources*. Plenum Press, New York.

2 Anaesthesia for CO_2 laser surgery

A. C. WAINWRIGHT

The brevity of surgical laryngoscopy belies the dangers and difficulties of the anaesthetic. The combination of the extreme surgical stimulus; the poor general health of the majority of adult patients and the sharing of the airway, all conspire to create these problems. As if these were not enough, the presence of the CO_2 laser adds new dangers. The complicating factors will be discussed first in order that the logic for and against the various techniques may be understood.

2.1 The surgical requirements

The surgeon requires a clear view of a still larynx with access for any operative measures that he may need to perform, and the time to do them (Carruth *et al.*, 1986).

2.2 The surgical stimulus

The surgical stimulus causes a combined rise in both pulse rate and arterial pressure; the latter caused by arteriolar constriction (Davies, Cronin and Cowie, 1981; Prys-Roberts, 1980). This combined rise causes a marked increase in cardiac workload. Patients who have hypertension even if treated show a greater rise in vascular resistance (Davies, Cronin and Cowie, 1981; Prys-Roberts, 1980).

2.3 General health of adult patients

Although there will be a proportion of patients with a benign or traumatic aetiology, the majority of adult patients who present for laryngoscopy are long-standing smokers of cigarettes. These patients

Anaesthesia for CO_2 laser surgery

will have widespread atheroma, the presence of which should be assumed so that complications are searched for diligently. In particular, the adequacy of the coronary, cerebral and renal circulations should be checked as well as the extent and efficacy of any treatment for hypertension. The problem for the anaesthetist, therefore, is to limit the effects of the increase in workload on an ischaemic and already overloaded heart and circulation. The principal choice lies between inhalational agents and drugs acting more specifically on the cardiovascular system. These fall into two groups, namely those that are longer acting and the shorter acting, that are generally more difficult to administer as they require to be given by infusion. The first group includes both the beta blockers and the vasodilators, such as pentolinium and hydralazine. The shorter acting include sodium nitroprusside, trimetaphan and intravenous nitrates. The choice will depend on the condition of the patient, the likely length of the operation and the potential problems of any unopposed long-acting drugs post-operatively.

Respiratory disease is a second major problem that must be borne in mind and suitably allowed for in determining the choice of anaesthesia. Chronic obstructive airways disease will, in particular, make ventilation difficult and may be a contra-indication to some of the techniques mentioned later if sufficiently severe. Any form of respiratory disease is an indication for an increase in inspired oxygen over that of room air. This affects the anaesthetic choice when the CO_2 laser is being used as it alters the flammability of other materials.

There are many other diseases which may alter the choice of anaesthetic but only a few will be mentioned. Obesity will make artificial ventilation more difficult and anatomical variations may cause difficulties of access.

Any situation where the airway is shared will inevitably cause difficulties for both surgeon and anaesthetist. It is essential therefore for there to be close cooperation between them with each appreciating the other's difficulties.

2.4 Complications of the CO_2 laser

The extra difficulty that the CO_2 laser adds to work in the larynx is flammability. Although the tissues are only heated to 100°C, plastics and rubbers are heated at a rate of about 5000°C/s. Any increase in the level of oxygen will increase flammability as will nitrous oxide. It should not be forgotten that although nitrous oxide is pharmacologically inert, it is chemically unstable and supports combustion slightly better than oxygen (Leonard, 1975; Chilcoat, Byles and Kellman, 1983).

Techniques with adults

Helium has been shown to reduce the flammability (Pashayan and Gravenstein, 1985). It should also be remembered that oxygen does not burn, it only supports combustion of other chemicals.

There has been discussion about the desirability of red-rubber versus PVC in relation to their relative flammabilities (Hermens, Bennett and Hirshman 1983): PVC ignites more easily. But this discussion is irrelevant as the only acceptable standard is that neither be allowed to ignite.

2.5 Techniques with adults

The fact that there are various techniques suggests that none of them is perfect. There are three basic types: (1) a standard endotracheal tube suitably protected; (2) a specially designed endotracheal tube; (3) using no endotracheal tube at all.

2.5.1 A STANDARD ENDOTRACHEAL TUBE SUITABLY PROTECTED

As mentioned above, there is some discussion as to whether it is safer to use a PVC endotracheal tube or a red-rubber tube. The author uses PVC for the reasons stated above and because red-rubber tubes are easier to kink and have thicker walls. If a PVC tube is used then the best one is a microlaryngeal tube as it provides a better view of the larynx with adequate artificial ventilation.

Whichever tube is used, it must be protected from the laser. There are several ways of wrapping the tube to protect it. The oldest and best is to use 12 mm (0.5 in) aluminium tape. This is (Figures 2.1 and 2.2) wound round spirally starting at the cuff and working upwards for about 10–12 cm (4–5 in.). It must be started at the distal end in order that the laser beam does not get under the edge. As it is wound round there must be just enough overlap for the same reason, but not too much or the tape will acquire creases. It is better to use 12 mm as opposed to 25 mm tape. There is a temptation to stick the 25 mm tape longitudinally down the length of the tube. This should be resisted as it will make the tube even more likely to kink. The spirally wound wrapping has a small amount of movement in it which helps to reduce the tendency to kink. About 12 cm of wrapping is enough to cover the length of the tube at risk for laryngeal lesions without covering that part of the tube which curves more sharply in the oropharynx where kinking is most likely to occur.

Other materials that have been suggested include moistened gauze and silver foil. Moistened gauze is both bulky and more difficult to stick

Anaesthesia for CO_2 laser surgery

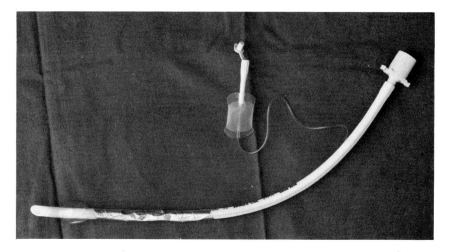

Figure 2.1 Microlaryngeal tube (5.0 mm) wrapped with aluminium tape.

firmly to the tube; it must be kept wet at all times. Silver foil is the silvered end to recording tape. Not only is this too thin, but it is also laminated to plastic and therefore of no benefit at all.

The principal advantage of a wrapped endotracheal tube is in the patient who is difficult to ventilate because of either obesity or lung disease. It also allows the surgeon to protect the trachea when lesions on the edge of the cords are being treated as he may put a wet swab between the cuff and the cords. In practice it is probable that damage to the trachea in these cases is not as relevant as was thought. It is important to stress that the cuff must always be protected with a wet swab or pledgelet. It is also advisable to fill the cuff with saline so that

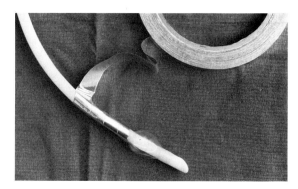

Figure 2.2 Correct method of wrapping.

Techniques with adults

puncturing of the cuff will be quickly noted and it will help to extinguish any tendency to combustion of the cuff. Vourc'h, Tannieres and Frêche (1979) pointed out that the tube should not be securely adhered to the patient so that in the event of fire it may be more rapidly removed.

The disadvantages of the wrapped tube are (1) the tendency to kink, (2) the sharp edge of the tape and (3) the reduction of the surgical visual field. As mentioned above a wrapped tube becomes liable to kink where it is wrapped. Attention to detail of the wrapping reduces this tendency, but it is nevertheless likely to occur. Although it is essential to make sure that any tube in the surgical field is properly covered any further covering is liable to kinkage where the curves are sharp. The sharp edges are liable to damage the vocal cords as they pass through. These two considerations also prevent the passage of the tube through the nose. Any tube will tend to reduce the extent of the surgical field. The relevance will depend on the position of the lesion requiring treatment.

2.5.2 SPECIALLY DESIGNED TUBES IN ADULTS

The first successful specially designed tube was that of Norton and DeVos (1978). This is made of stainless steel, is very flexible and has the

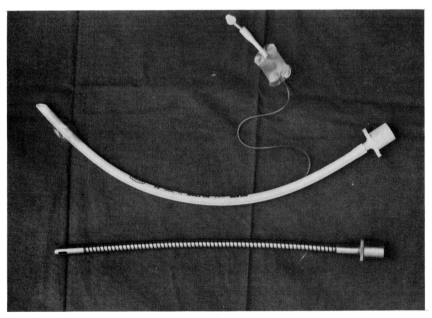

Figure 2.3 5.0 mm Microlaryngeal tube and Norton tube.

Anaesthesia for CO_2 laser surgery

over-riding advantage that it is completely laser proof. On the other hand it has (Figure 2.3) no cuff and it has a thick wall so that a tube that is thin enough to allow good access to the cords is too small for the patient to be able to breath through. For this reason it is not used as much as its degree of laser resistance might suggest. Its principal use is likely to be in patients who cannot be ventilated with the Sanders injector, though there are new developments with the high frequency jet ventilator that may make even this use outdated (Herbert, Berlin and Eberle, 1985; Smith, 1985).

Another kind of special tube that is available is the silicon tube (Gaba, Hayes and Goode, 1984), which has the advantage that in the presence of heat silicon dioxide is formed which is particularly heat and flame resistant. Silicon tube is available either as a 5.0 mm cuffed tube with aluminium paste on the outside or with two cuffs or a wire coil in the wall. As penetration of the tube is unlikely to occur in air because of the silicon dioxide, in air it is virtually laser proof. Unfortunately as soon as the oxygen concentration of the gas rises it becomes flammable (Figure 2.4). When ignition occurs the tube burns as freely as PVC and unlike the latter is not self extinguishing when the oxygen is removed. The precise oxygen concentration is not yet known but is being investigated. Until further data become available it is suggested that the maximum concentration used is 25% which effectively means air. It

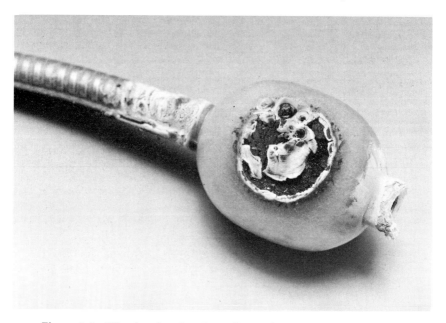

Figure 2.4 Silastic tube showing effects of combustion with laser.

Techniques with adults

remains for the anaesthetist to decide whether he feels that each patient is best anaesthetized using air mixtures or whether oxygen enrichment is preferred in view of the respiratory and cardiovascular state of that patient. Helium has been shown to have a marked effect on flammability and should be considered as an alternative carrier gas where higher concentrations of oxygen are required (Pashayan and Gravenstein, 1985).

Extensive work has been carried out in Southampton to try to perfect a tube made of non-flammable plastic by protecting it with a thin layer of either aluminium or silver or gold to produce a tube that is both laser proof and has all the desirable qualities that one expects from the modern plastic endotracheal tube. So far this has been insufficiently successful to market but work is still progressing (Russell, 1984).

2.5.3 NO ENDOTRACHEAL TUBE IN ADULTS

This is synonymous in adults with jet ventilation. The most widely used form of jet ventilation is the Sanders injector. This is also the most satisfactory method of delivering general anaesthesia to adult patients when the CO_2 laser is being used in the larynx. It is used in much the same way as in bronchoscopy. Since the normal surgical laryngoscope is tubular, provided the tip of the laryngoscope is at or near the larynx, adequate ventilation can be achieved. It has the advantages that it is totally laser proof, it provides the surgeon with a totally unobstructed view of the larynx, and it is not traumatic to the vocal cords. Anaesthesia will need to be provided intravenously using a combination of adequate depth of anaesthesia to control the cardiovascular responses as mentioned on p. 35 and muscle relaxation to keep the cords still and yet allow rapid recovery. Propofol would seem particularly suitable as it combines a marked lack of cumulative effect, with a degree of hypotension.

The principal disadvantages are the difficulty in achieving adequate ventilation in the obese and those with more severe levels of lung disease, and the risk of causing surgical emphysema (Steward and Fearon, 1981, 1982; Oliverio, Ruder and Abramson, 1981; Scamman and McCabe, 1984; Glesnki et al., 1985). The second problem is most likely to be caused by using an extension to the injector which is both of small diameter and protrudes beyond the laryngoscope. An injector of larger size with a smooth end such as the Norton tube is less likely to cause this kind of trauma. The alternative in this particular group of patients is to use a wrapped tube in spite of its other disadvantages. An injector end which does not protrude but gives a good flow gives the best

Anaesthesia for CO_2 laser surgery

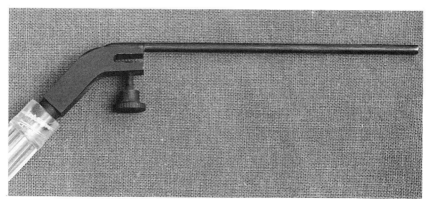

Figure 2.5 Downs-Carruth modification of Sanders injector.

characteristics with the Sanders injector (Figures 2.5 and 2.6). An alternative tubing is malleable copper tubing (Herbert, Berlin and Eberle, 1985). This sort of tubing is likely to come into its own with the form of ventilation that is still being tried out but is likely to prove the

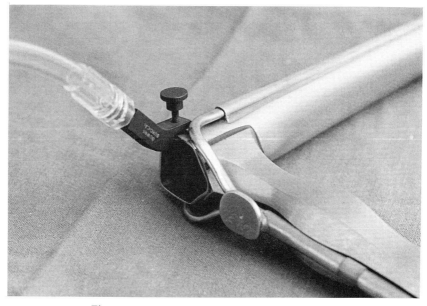

Figure 2.6 Injector attached to laryngoscope.

best in terms of satisfactory ventilation in all patients, both the obese and those with severe respiratory obstruction, and in its overall safety. This is the use of the high-frequency jet ventilation which for an adult only requires an inlet tube of 1.2 mm internal diameter and an outlet airway of 6 mm^2 (Smith, 1985). Since it is unlikely that any adult with an airway of less than 6 mm^2 would reach the anaesthetist alive it is suitable for any adult patient. The inlet tube may not only be placed in the larynx using a tube such as that from Vienna, but it may be placed through the cricothyroid membrane or even between rings of the trachea using a needle such as a Tuohy needle of about 14 guage size. It has the advantage of (a) being laser proof if the tube is made of metal, (b) providing adequate ventilation in patients with pulmonary disease who may not be as suitable for other techniques, (c) providing good access and (d) being better for patients with obstructing lesions. For these reasons it may become the recommended technique in the future.

2.6 Patients with a tracheostomy

These patients should be anaesthetized using a metal tracheostomy tube such as the Negus silver tracheostomy tube. If a patient already has a fenestrated tube for speech it should be changed to the non-fenestrated variety prior to surgery and any connections from the anaesthetic circuit should be made of metal in order to make certain that there is no risk from heating of the connection or from inadvertent failure to change the tube (Carruth *et al.*, 1986; Wainwright, Moody and Carruth, 1981; Spargo, Van de Spek and Norton, 1986).

2.7 Lesions in the mouth

These present little problem. Either a PVC or a red-rubber tube of a normal size should be used suitably protected with 12 mm aluminium tape. A metal connector should be used. If the lesion is on the anterior two thirds of the tongue or the anterior part of the mouth, the tube may be wrapped from about 3 cm above the cuff so that enough of the tube is protected but the sharp edges of the aluminium tape do not actually pass through the vocal cords. Any suitable general anaesthetic technique may be used suited to the patient. If there is any doubt about how far back the lesion spreads then the tube should be wrapped from the cuff and the cuff protected as though a laryngeal lesion were being treated.

2.8 Paediatric patients

Many of the paediatric patients who present for CO_2 laser surgery to the larynx are children aged approximately 2 years old with viral papillomata in the larynx. There are basically two methods which are used. The first is the use of the Sanders injector in very much the same way as in the adult. Various authors have suggested that this is a highly dangerous technique because of the larger risk of surgical emphysema (Steward and Fearon, 1981, 1982; Oliverio, Ruder and Abramson, 1981; Scamman and McCabe, 1984), and that it is therefore unacceptable. Never the less it is still used with success. In any event, care should be taken to remove this risk.

The alternative technique is to use spontaneous ventilation under deep inhalational anaesthesia. Halothane is the most widely used as depth is required. Enflurane is not suitable because of the high pCO_2 generated at depth. The risks of cerebral irritation also make it an unsuitable agent. When the child is deep enough to tolerate surgical stimulation of the larynx, a catheter is passed into the nose having first been marked at about 3–4 cm from the tip. This mark is to make sure that the tip of the tube does not protrude from under the soft palate. Oxygen and halothane are then blown at the larynx down the tube with the child continuing to breath spontaneously throughout the procedure. It is important to get the child deep enough before surgery commences as in the author's experience it requires 3% halothane to maintain adequate depth. The other advantage of this method is that even where a hole for respiration through the diseased larynx may not be apparent, respiration continues without the need to produce an airway surgically as may happen if the injector is being used where paralysis is required. A high flow of gas should be used to make sure that during expiration any cinders are not blown back onto the catheter causing ignition as has been reported (Hirshman and Smith, 1980).

In no branch of anaesthesia is it more applicable than anaesthesia for CO_2 laser to the larynx to say 'Where the consequences of error are certain to be disastrous it is hardly possible to be too careful'.

References

Carruth, J. A. S., Morgan, N. J., Mielsen, M. S., Phillips, J. J. and Wainwright, A. C. (1986), The treatment of laryngeal stenosis using the CO_2 laser. *Clin. Otolaryngol.*, **11**, 145–8.

Chilcoat, R. T., Byles, P. H. and Kellman, R. M. (1983), The hazards of nitrous oxide during laser endoscopic surgery. *Anesthesiology*, **59**, 258.

References

Davies, M. J., Cronin, K. D. and Cowie, R. W. (1981) The prevention of hypertension at intubation. *Anesthesia*, **36**, 147–52.

Gaba, D. M., Hayes, D. M. and Goode, R. L. (1984), Incendiary characteristics of a new laser resistant endotracheal tube. *Anesthesiology*, **61**, A417.

Glenski, J. A., MacKenzie, R. A., Maragos, N. E. and Southorn, P. A. (1985), Assessing tidal volume and detecting hyperinflation during Ventari jet ventilation for microlaryngeal surgery. *Anesthesiology*, **63**, 554–7.

Herbert, J. T., Berlin, I. and Eberle, R. (1985), Jet ventilation via a copper endotracheal tube for CO_2 laser surgery of the cropharynx. *Laryngoscope*, **95**, 1276–7.

Hermens, J. M., Bennett, M. J. and Hirshman, C. A. (1983) Anesthesia for laser surgery. *Anesth Analg.*, **62**, 218–29.

Hirshman, C. A. and Smith, J. (1980), Indirect ignition of the endotracheal tube during carbon dioxide laser surgery. *Arch. Otolaryngol.* **106**, 639–41.

Leonard, P. F. (1975), The lower limits of flammability of halothane, enflurane and isoflurane. *Anesth. Analg.* **54**, 238–40.

Norton, M. L. and DeVos, P. (1978), A new endotracheal tube for laser surgery of the larynx. *Ann. Otol. Rhinol. Laryngol.*, **87**, 554–7.

Oliverio, R. M., Ruder, C. B. and Abramson, A. L. (1981), Jet ventilation for laryngeal microsurgery. *Br. J. Anaesth.*, **53**, 1010.

Pashayan, A. G. and Gravenstein, J. S. (1985), Helium retards endotracheal tube fires from carbon dioxide lasers. *Anesthesiology*, **62**, 274–7.

Prys-Roberts, C. (1980), in *The Circulation in Anaesthesia*. (ed. C. Prys-Roberts), Blackwell Scientific Publications, Oxford, p. 135.

Russell, C. R. (1984), Tracheal tubes for laser surgery. *Anaesthesia*, **39**, 293–4.

Scamman, F. L. and McCabe, B. F. (1984), Evaluation of supraglottic jet ventilation for laser surgery of the larynx. *Anesthesiology*, **61**, A447.

Smith, B. E. (1985), The penlon bromsgrove high frequency jet ventilator for adult and paediatric use. *Anaesthesia*, **40**, 790–6.

Spargo, P. M., Van de Spek, A. F. L. and Norton, M. L. (1986), Lasers in medicine: The physics of lasers and implications for the anesthesiologist. Personal communication.

Steward, D. J. and Fearon, B. (1981), Anaesthesia for laryngoscopy. *Br. J. Anaesth.*, **53**, 320.

Steward, D. J. and Fearon, B. (1982), Laryngeal microsurgery. *Br. J. Anaesth.*, **54**, 364.

Vourc'h, G., Tannieres, M. L. and Frêche, G. (1979), Anaesthesia for microsurgery of the larynx using the carbon dioxide laser. *Anaesthesia*, **34**, 53–7.

Wainwright, A. C., Moody, R. A. and Carruth, J. A. S. (1981), Anaesthetic safety with the CO_2 laser. *Anaesthesia*, **36**, 411–15.

3 The laser in laryngeal disease

GEORGE T. SIMPSON

3.1 Introduction

The intention of this chapter, is to provide a comprehensive overview of the current use of lasers in laryngology. This approach presents specific technical guidelines for laser surgery, but also reflects our philosophy in the management of a variety of laryngeal problems. The discussion is a synthesis of the combined laser surgical experience of the members of the Department of Otolaryngology at Boston University School of Medicine (including M. Stuart Strong, Geza Jako, Charles W. Vaughan, Gerald B. Healy, Stanley M. Shapshay, Graeme A. McDonald, and George T. Simpson). While some may differ from my techniques, philosophy or suggestions, the combined laser surgical experience of our Department represents several thousand surgical procedures. From this perspective, the current concepts of the role of laser techniques in the management of laryngeal diseases are described.

The introduction of the CO_2 laser has revolutionized laryngeal surgery. The laser allows increased surgical precision that is an order of magnitude above that of traditional endolaryngeal surgery. Operations formerly performed only by external procedures can now be performed endoscopically with minimal morbidity or hospitalization. It must always be kept in mind, however, that the laser is a surgical instrument and only a part of a complete surgical system. A number of factors are important in allowing successful and effective laryngeal laser surgery. Essential components of effective laser endolaryngeal surgery include effective general anaesthesia, wide exposure of the operative field, a magnified view, adequate time for a performance of an unhurried procedure, and special instrumentation.

3.2 Anaesthesia (Norton, 1983)

Endolaryngeal surgery requires complete patient immobility and safety. These requirements mandate general anaesthesia with complete muscular paralysis, physiological monitoring, and a secure airway. Complete and effective communication between the surgeon and the anaesthesiologist are essential before and during surgery. Each must thoroughly understand the other's problems, techniques, resources and repertoire. This will usually forestall problems but will also enhance effective response to unexpected complications. Both the surgeon and the anaesthesiologist must always keep in mind that cardiac arrhythmias are a common response to laryngeal stimulation and are usually temporary and without permanent effect. Adequate pre-operative and intra-operative medication is essential to minimize these problems. With proper planning and effective communication virtually all problems can be prevented or minimized.

3.3 Exposure of the operating field

Wide exposure of the operating field is important in any surgery but is essential in endolaryngeal surgery. In the past, this was provided by the Lynch suspension system. This system is complicated to use and does not retract the endotracheal tube out of the operating field. It has been largely superseded by other methods of laryngeal exposure. A number of wide-angle laryngoscopes have been developed specifically for microscopic laryngeal surgery. These are wide enough to allow binocular vision with the operating microscope for depth perception and to allow adequate room for bimanual surgery with a variety of instruments. Each of these laryngoscopes differs slightly in configuration and each offers advantages. None is perfect for every case. The surgeon must select the largest laryngoscope the patient can accept as well as the one that best exposes the area of disease.

The Jako-Kleinsasser laryngoscopes have a wide posterior configuration and provide an excellent view of the posterior larynx. The width may be too wide, however, to allow an adequate view of the anterior commissure. The Dedo laryngoscope is narrower overall with a configuration similar to the Holinger anterior commissure laryngoscope and usually provides excellent exposure of the anterior commissure. The Lynch suspension apparatus is too complicated for routine use and has the additional disadvantage of not retracting the endotracheal tube out of the operating field. The surgeon must select the laryngoscope most suitable for particular application which allows complete visual-

Exposure of the operating field

ization of the lesion. It may be necessary to change laryngoscopes one or more times during the procedure. Occasionally other methods may be necessary in unusual situations. Dingman and Crow-Davis mouth-gags may allow exposure of the epiglottis in certain situations. These should be supported on a stand or other suspension unit as for tonsillectomy.

Illumination is essential for surgery and this requires a distal light source. Standard fibreoptic cables and lights are suitable for most procedures but when photographic documentation is required, a Xenon or other high intensity light source providing 500 W of light energy is necessary and must be delivered through a larger than normal fibreoptic cable. When taking photographs the microscope light should be turned off since it tends to reflect off the laryngoscope and interfere rather than aid vision and photography. Suspension systems are an essential component of the laryngoscopic system. Laryngoscopic suspension is essential for all microscopic laryngeal surgery especially that utilizing the laser. This suspension allows both hands to be free to perform surgical procedures. The Lewy-Kleinsasser systems work well when the larynx can be exposed. However, they require hyperextension of the neck and this may make laryngeal exposure more difficult. If the suspension system is placed on the chest respiratory movements negate

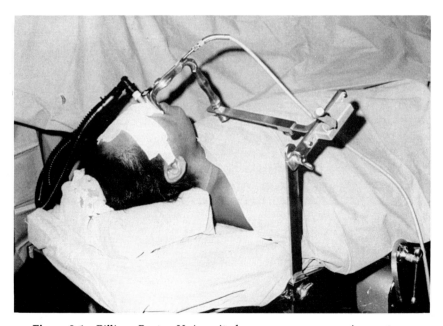

Figure 3.1 Pilling–Boston University laryngoscope suspension system.

The laser in laryngeal disease

the precision of the laser surgical system. The Jackson-Boyce sniffing position with the neck flexed and the head extended provides ideal exposure of the larynx for surgery (Jackson and Jackson, 1945). The Pilling–Boston University system is a true suspension system for laryngeal surgery (Figure 3.1). The suspension forces are directed away from the teeth and gums and the force vectors are centred on the larynx. The table can be repositioned without requiring resuspension. There is no movement of the suspension system with respiration and the larynx and trachea are in a good alignment for use of a Venturi ventilation system.

3.4 Adequate time for unhurried surgery

Precision microsurgery requires unhurried technique. Anatomy and pathology can be carefully assessed and delicate procedures can be carefully performed. A major factor in allowing for sufficient time is adequate general anaesthesia with complete muscular relaxation. Inadvertent and unanticipated patient movements are bothersome during any surgical procedure but can be extremely hazardous in microscopic lasery surgery. Adequate time is necessary to allow processing and examination of frozen section biopsy sections. If further biopsies are necessary these can be easily performed if the patient is still at an adequate plane of anaesthesia.

3.5 Magnification

A standard binocular size microscope should be equipped with straight eye pieces and 20× oculars which provide a larger image while retaining adequate depth of focus. Most microscopic laryngeal surgery is performed at the 10× or 16× setting. Careful examination of a specific lesion or wound bed requires 25× or even 40× magnification. A 400 mm front lens allows adequate working distance between the microscope and laryngoscope. This allows for binocular vision through the laryngoscope and enough room to manoeuvre surgical instruments.

3.6 Special instruments (Andrews and Baim, 1982)

A number of instruments and other materials are essential for microscopic laryngeal laser surgery. The microscopic laryngeal instruments such as miniaturized alligator and cup forceps, probes, and scissors are basically otological instruments with 22 cm handles. These have been developed for use through laryngoscopes. Other essential instruments include microlaryngeal suction tips which have a significantly smaller diameter than the usual suction tips and also have a finger hole, for controlling the amount of suction. Double-lumen suction irrigator tips are helpful for supravital staining of laryngeal lesions. Andrews anterior commissure retractors (cord protectors) have several uses including protecting the anterior end of one vocal fold while surgery is performed on the other fold or in the anterior commissure (this prevents web formation during healing). A suction channel allows smoke evacuation. The cord protector can be used for separating the cords for subglottic surgical work and to enhance respiratory flow with use of the Venturi system. Surgical mirrors which are either of solid steel or have a metallic front face allow delivery of a reflected beam to the subglottic area. A suction cautery tip can be invaluable. Rubber tooth protectors are important when suspension laryngoscopy is performed. Additional suction tips can be placed alongside a laryngoscope or in one of the light channels of the laryngoscope to evacuate smoke and steam, thereby enhancing visibility and preventing heat damage to surrounding tissue. Small neurosurgical cottonoids soaked in saline are placed below the vocal folds and over the endotracheal tube cuff to protect it from penetration by the laser beam. The attached cotton thread allows easy removal. Reinforced silastic sheeting for custom fabrication of rolled stents and keels should be available. Suture material including 3 and 4-0 chromic suture with small needles can be used in suturing mucosal flaps. Heavy nylon (0,2-0 and 3-0) can be used for the percutaneous anchoring of stents and keels. Woven stainless-steel suture such as is used for pacemakers can also be used similarly. Desiccated slices of cucumber, stored in absolute alcohol, are used to mount biopsy specimens. Tolidine blue 0 dye is painted on epithelial tissue for vital staining to help identify atypia and malignancy (Strong and Vaughan, 1970). This will be discussed in further detail below.

3.7 Safety (Davis and Simpson, 1983; Healy 1983)

Details of safety procedures for use in laser surgery are given in Chapter 1. The surgeon as well as other personnel must guarantee the safety of both the patient and other operating room personnel. This is a vital consideration in laser surgery. Fire is the greatest single hazard. No flammable materials should be used in the operating field where they could be contacted and ignited by the laser unless they are soaked with saline or water. Wet cotton eyepads are placed and secured with wet

The laser in laryngeal disease

cloth tape to protect the eyes. The face is covered with a wet cloth towel during use of the laser. In endolaryngeal surgery there is the danger that endotracheal tubes can be ignited on impact of the laser in a high oxygen atmosphere; nitrous oxide also supports combustion. In multiple tests in our laboratory we have determined that PVC tubes are especially hazardous. Newly available laser-resistant tubes of silicone can burn and produce silicone ash which is very adherent to the mucosa; we do not recommend them. The safest tube to use is the flexible metal Norton endotracheal tube but these are not widely available, can occasionally be traumatic to laryngeal mucosa, and are difficult to insert. We believe that overall red-rubber endotracheal tubes are the most practical for regular use (Figure 3.2). On laser impact the rubber tends to melt rather than burn. The tube should be wrapped with metallic foil tape (3M, Radio Shack) and care should be taken that this is truly metallic foil and not a mylar tape containing metal fragments as such tape can burn. The tape is wrapped on the tube in a direction from distal to proximal overlapping each turn by one half the width of the previous turn. This allows tube flexion without exposing the underlying tube to possible laser impact. Tincture of Benzoin solution sprayed or painted on the tube provides added adhesion for the metallic foil tape. Ideally the resistance to ignition of the tube to be used after wrapping with metallic tape should be ascertained prior to the start of each operation. We inflate the endotracheal tube balloon cuff with saline. In children an endotracheal tube without a cuff should be used. The endotracheal tube cuff is further protected with wet neurosurgical cottonoids placed over the cuff below the vocal folds. Another hazard, especially to the patient, comes from misdirection of the laser beam. Harm can be prevented by assuring that the face and eyes are completely covered with wet cotton eye pads and a wet towel cloth. All operating room personnel should wear eyeglasses or appropriate goggles for eye protection against the reflected beam. If a Neodymium-YAG laser is used, appropriate filtering lenses in the goggles are necessary. Another source of potential patient injury comes from use of an inappropriate power density in the laser beam and from excessive duration of application of the beam. Excessive heat absorption and conduction can produce excessive fibrosis and scarring.

If a fire occurs, the endotracheal tube (if burning) must be removed immediately. The tube and any other burning materials are immersed in a basin of water to extinguish the fire. Such a basin must be prepared in advance and kept on a side table for possible use. The patient is ventilated with 100% O_2 delivered by mask. The surgeon examines the entire airway with a laryngoscope and bronchoscope and any airway ash is removed. An airway is secured. If any airway injury is detected

Postoperative care

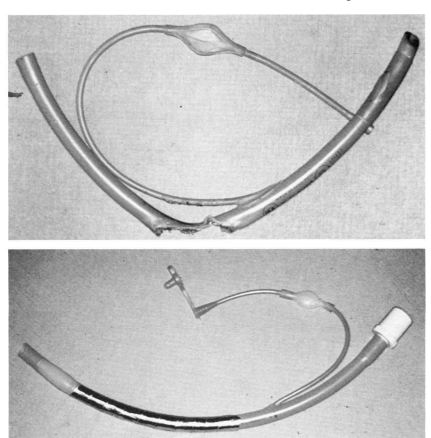

Figure 3.2 Endotracheal tube protection. (A) Red rubber endotracheal tube impacted by CO_2 laser in 100% oxygen smoulders and melts without explosive ignition. (B) Metallic foil-wrapped red-rubber endotracheal tube after laser impact in 100% oxygen with no effect.

intravenous antibiotic must be administered. Steroids are given to all patients. Patients should be carefully monitored in an intensive care setting and the pulmonary and airway status carefully observed.

3.8 Postoperative care

Voice rest is commonly prescribed in the postoperative period. This is usually interpreted to mean no talking, whispering, shouting, etc. while relying upon written messages. It is virtually impossible to

The laser in laryngeal disease

maintain this degree of voice rest and is in fact unrealistic. Unstressed, soft relaxed, higher pitched vocalization with a breathy quality because of air escape is not traumatic and will aid return of vocal function minimizing oedema formation and aiding its resolution. Shouting and whispering are forbidden because of the forced glottic closure necessary for either. The voice should only be used for necessary communication and in the manner described. When patients have worked with a competent voice therapist preoperatively, and have learned the fundamentals of normal voice production and use their voice gently, they will have minimal postoperative complications. In more extensive surgery, hoarseness may persist for two to four weeks, but in general the voice is normal within three or four days after surgery.

The airway must be carefully monitored in the immediate postoperative period. Adults should have adequate humidification of inspired air using a mask. Humidification should be a cool mist. Infants and children do best in a croup tent. Humidification is maintained overnight. In general, laryngeal airway oedema has been minimized by following this programme. In addition, all patients receive dexamethasone (1 g kg to a maximum of 20 mg) in the immediate preoperative period to suppress oedema formation or progression.

Suspension laryngoscopy may effect the cardiac regulatory mechanism and produce arrhythmias potentially resulting in myocardial infarction (Strong *et al.*, 1974). All patients over forty or with cardiac risk factors should have an electrocardiogram following surgery. If changes from the preoperative electrocardiogram are present careful monitoring with serial electrocardiograms and enzyme determinations must be performed.

On the day following surgery the patient is comfortable with normal alimentation and a voice suitable for necessary communication. Analgesics are usually unnecessary. Antibiotics are used only in the presence of a tracheotomy or laryngeal stent.

3.9 Major surgery for specific benign organic lesions

3.9.1 VOCAL NODULES

Nodules on the vocal folds presents as thickening in the midportion of the mobile cord at approximately the junction of the anterior and middle thirds. The nodules form in response to the mechanical trauma or friction from rubbing against the other cord or an opposing nodule. The earliest response to this irritation is the accumulation of oedema fluid (a blister) in Reinke's space. Without further irritation this will

Specific benign organic lesions

resolve in 48 h. If the mechanical trauma persists an inflammatory response develops with increased vascularity and oedema. This is reversible until fibrosis develops. A fibrotic nodule is no longer amenable to medical measures or voice therapy. The fibrosis causes contraction of the nodule and fixation to the underlying tissue.

Vocal nodules may have a deleterious effect on the voice. The unique vocal quality in many professional 'popular' singers results from nodules. These should not be tampered with by the surgeon. One-third of operatic sopranos and tenors have nodules without obvious detriment in vocal quality (Lancina, 1972).

Voice therapy is effective in resolving most nodules. Anti-inflammatory medicines mask the inflammatory response and do not prevent damage or further progression of the problem. They are rarely indicated and in general should be avoided.

Surgical removal of nodules should be considered if there is no improvement in response to voice therapy, the diagnosis is uncertain and excision is required, or a fibrotic nodule is observed.

The surgical technique involves vaporization of the nodule. This is simple, direct and effective and is followed by prompt healing. The laser beam is used to shave the nodule off the vocal cord. Wet neurosurgical cottonoids are placed below the vocal fold to protect the endotracheal tube and subglottic area. The laser beam is aimed onto the wet cottonoid and is gradually moved onto the edge of the nodule. A short, high-powered burst is used for vaporization. The nodule is shaved to the appropriate level in Reinke's space. A small depression remains, but this should not extend into the vocal ligament. This will rapidly epithialize.

Post-operatively the patient requires cool mist inhalations. No antibiotics or aspirin are used. Mild analgesics are all that is necessary. The patient assumes a normal diet and communicates with a gentle voice. An electrocardiogram is obtained when indicated. The patient is discharged the following day to continue on voice therapy in the future.

3.9.2 POLYPOID VOCAL FOLD LESIONS (Figure 3.3)

Polypoid vocal fold lesions represent oedema in Reinke's space. They involve one or both cords and occur for unknown reasons. The typical patient is a middle-aged, female smoker with a long history of patterns of vocal abuse.

Oedema fluid collects in the loose alveolar tissue of the vocal cord between the anterior commissure and the vocal process. This oedema occurs predominantly on the superior surface of the cord and stops subglottically at the junction of the squamous and respiratory

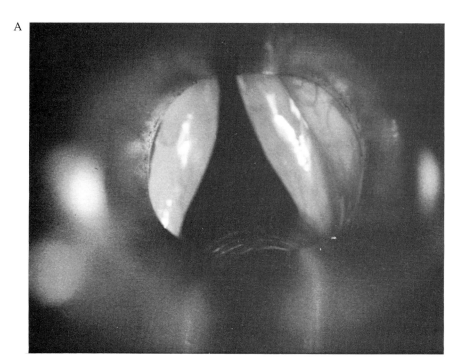

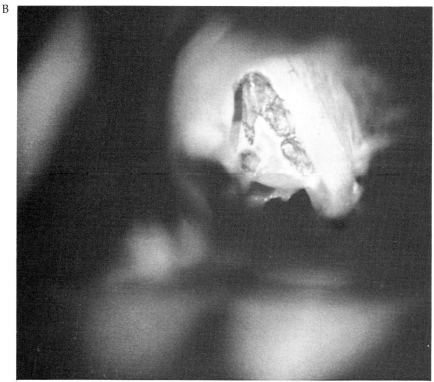

Specific benign organic lesions

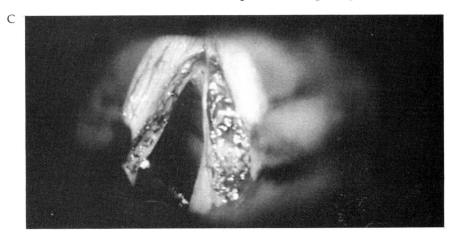

Figure 3.3 Polypoid vocal fold lesions: (A) polypoid vocal folds; (B) excision under tension; (C) post excision.

epithelium. As the oedema fluid accumulates it gradually increases in size to form a wide-based polyp. Vocal pitch decreases and greater force is required to produce sound.

The most effective treatment is voice therapy, but this may not be completely effective and if the patient desires improvement in the voice, surgery may be necessary. It is absolutely essential that the patient stops smoking. If the patient cannot eliminate this habit, surgery should not be considered as the problem will recur. The patient must be warned of the necessity of elevating the pitch of their voice after surgery and that there will be a period of vocal roughness or hoarseness for a period of time after surgery.

The surgical technique includes the usual safety precautions mentioned above. The polypoid area to be removed is outlined with the laser with an initial cut beginning 1–2 mm posterior to the anterior commissure. A second cut is created posteriorly to the polyp. The lesion is grasped with cup forceps and retracted medially. An incision is made from anterior to posterior on the superior surface of the vocal fold while medial traction is maintained on the cord. The polyp is dissected from the underlying vocalis muscle, taking care not to damage the muscle. This creates a large denuded area which will result in ulceration which will require several weeks to heal before full epithelialization has occurred. An alternative technique involves incising the superior surface of the vocal fold mucosa and aspirating or vaporizing the oedematous areolar contents overlying the vocalis muscle and vocal ligament.

The laser in laryngeal disease

The excess mucosa is then retracted superiorly and excised. Fibrinogen tissue glue or endolaryngeal suture is used to approximate the mucosa.

3.9.3 VOCAL FOLD POLYPS (Figure 3.4)

Sessile (broad-based) polyps can be treated in similar fashion as polypoid changes. The pedunculated (narrow-based) polyps occur at, or anterior to, the midportion of the vocal fold. There is a history of severe vocal abuse which leads to sudden hoarseness. Frequently a subepithelial haemorrhage is present. The cycle of recurrent vocal abuse and haemorrhage leads to granulation tissue formation and a development

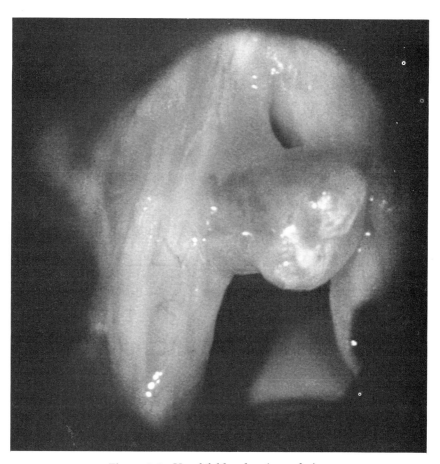

Figure 3.4 Vocal fold polyp (vascular).

Specific benign organic lesions

of a polyp with multiple vascular channels and oedematous matrix. The polyp appears white and translucent but may be opaque red colour depending on its vascularity. There is usually a large feeding vessel.

The carbon dioxide is an ideal instrument for excising vascular polyps becaue of its haemostatic qualities. The polyp is grasped with a cup forcep, retracted medially and its stalk cut flush with the vocal fold surface. Any remaining granulation tissue is vaporized and the feeding vessel destroyed by laser photocoagulation.

3.9.4 VOCAL FOLD CYSTS (Figure 3.5)

Submucosal cysts may form in a supraglottic area or on the vocal fold, and possibly originate from minor salivary glands. Because minor salivary glands are rarely present in a true vocal fold, cysts are less common in this area. Examination shows a smooth rounded mass beneath a normal epithelium. A cyst occurring on the vocal fold produces a vocal disturbance. Cysts occurring elsewhere in the larynx may partially obstruct the airway or produce vocal muffling. Cysts of the vocal fold require careful dissection for complete removal as do cysts elsewhere in the body. This dissection is only possible with the latest generation of lasers having a beam spot size of 0.5 mm or less. This is necessary for delicate dissection. if such a laser instrument is unavailable, the cysts are best dissected for excision using conventional microsurgical techniques. Cysts occurring elsewhere in the larynx are marsupialized using the laser to unroof the cyst. The remaining cyst wall then provides epithelial coverage and rapid healing.

3.9.5 GRANULOMAS (Figure 3.6)

Granulomas form in response to repeated injury. Granulation tissue forms with the failure of scar tissue formation and the resultant failure of the normal re-establishment of epithelial coverage. When present in the vocal process area granulomas are frequently blamed on a history of endotracheal intubation and are even called 'intubation granulomas'. A careful history will frequently reveal the presence of a prolonged period of continued irritation particularly as a result of vocal abuse and gastro-oesophageal reflux.

Treatment of granulomas is non-surgical until an airway hazard develops or severe vocal disturbance occurs. Initial treatment is voice therapy with medical measures to control gastro-oesophageal reflux. Such measures include dietary alterations such as eliminating alcohol and tobacco, avoiding fluids with meals, more frequent smaller food

The laser in laryngeal disease

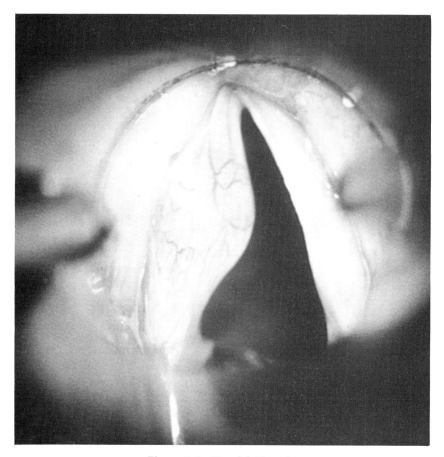

Figure 3.5 Vocal fold cyst.

portions, and avoidance of bedtime snacks or drinks. Elevating the head and shoulders in sleep may be beneficial and this may require the use of blocks or bricks under the legs at the head of the bed. Histamine antagonist medications such as ranitidine hydrochloride suppress baseline acid levels. This is particularly beneficial during sleep. If surgery is necessary to improve the airway or voice, the laser is used easily to excise the granuloma, coagulate any bleeding sites, and vaporize any residual granular tissue. Care must be taken to avoid exposure of cartilage particularly at the vocal process as this inhibits healing and promotes further granuloma formation.

Granulomas develop elsewhere in the larynx following injury or from infection. Surgical trauma including laser surgery can result in

Specific benign organic lesions

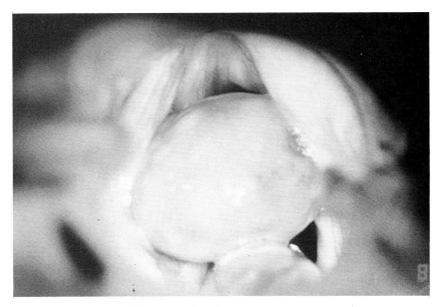

Figure 3.6 'Intubation' granuloma.

granuloma formation. Artificial materials such as stents and keels, while used specifically to prevent fibrotic adhesions, can also provoke granuloma formation.

Prevention is the best treatment for granulomas. Endotracheal tubes must be selected for proper size to prevent subglottic and posterior commissure necrosis and later granuloma formation. Stents and keels should be avoided unless absolutely necessary and then left in place for the minimal duration required and then removed. Antibiotics are used to prevent or treat laryngeal infections, and this minimizes or prevents formation of infectious granulomas. When granulomas persist and produce bothersome symptoms, they are easily vaporized with the laser.

3.9.6 CONTACT ULCERS

Contact ulcers develop over the vocal process at the arytenoid in response to harsh glottic closure. Actual ulceration is rarely present. These lesions are cup-shaped hypertrophic formations in the mucous membrane. Effective treatment consists of voice therapy. When there is a doubt as to the nature or aetiology of the lesion, excisional biopsy with the laser is helpful.

The laser in laryngeal disease

3.9.7 PAPILLOMAS (Strong et al., 1976; Simpson and Strong, 1983)

Papillomas are formed of branching stalks of connective tissue covered by histologically normal epithelium. It is now known that they occur in response to induction by one of several classes of papova viruses (Costa et al., 1981; Lack et al., 1980; Strauss and Jenson, 1985). Two basic manifestations occur: the simple and recurrent form.

Simple papillomas occur as isolated lesions and tend to be pedunculated with a stalk. They are occasionally found on the epiglottis, false vocal fold or aryepiglottic fold but rarely occur on the true vocal fold. They are also encountered on the palatine arch or uvula. The excision biopsy performed for diagnosis is usually curative. Thereafter the patient should be examined periodically to rule out recurrence.

3.9.8 RECURRENT RESPIRATORY PAPILLOMATOSIS (Strong et al., 1976; Simpson and Strong, 1983)

Recurrent respiratory papillomas can be found at virtually any site in the epithelium of the air passageways. They occur with particular frequency at points of constriction. As maximal cooling and drying of the surface occurs in these areas, ecological factors may favour expressions of the viral infection which may actually be present in widespread areas of epithelium. The glottis is the most frequent site of involvement, especially anteriorly. This disease occurs in all age groups with an equal incidence in both sexes. In the United States, the incidence is approximately seven cases per million per year or approximately 1500 new cases per year. Papilloma growth and recurrence are quite variable and unpredictable. Most frequent pattern is one of indolence requiring only infrequent surgical removal. In a few cases, however, recurrence is relentlessly aggressive and removals at intervals of two to three weeks may be necessary to maintain the airway. Papillomas may seem to disappear but this represents remission, only, as recurrences are common even after many years. Recurrences tend to occur in response to the stress of major illness, injury, surgery, or pregnancy.

As respiratory papillomatosis is a recurrent disease certain essential goals must be recognized. These include airway preservation, avoidance of dissemination, voice preservation and avoidance of other harm.

Airway preservation is the first and primary goal. As papillomas occur at the narrowest points in the airway they can be potentially life threatening especially in children. Mortality has been rare. The airway should be preserved with minimal trauma to avoid obstructive oedema, fibrosis, scarring, and ultimate stenosis.

Specific benign organic lesions

Avoidance of dissemination to other parts of the airway is a desirable goal. The single factor most obviously involved in dissemination is the tracheotomy. Its role is difficult to assess, however, as tracheotomy is required in the more aggressive forms of the disease with rapid recurrent airway obstruction at the laryngeal level, where tracheotomy can be life saving over a period of time. A tracheotomy, however, alters the ecology of the tracheobronchial tree by decreasing humidity and increasing cooling of the mucosal surfaces of the epithelial surfaces. If tracheotomy is necessary on an emergency basis, the patient should be decannulated as soon as a satisfactory and normal airway is established. Even when a few papillomas are present in the trachea, decannulation in association with laser vaporization usually will result in complete remission in the tracheal area. Interestingly papillomas are almost never seen below the glottic level and rarely even extend into the subglottic region unless a tracheotomy has been performed. From these factors one may surmise that this viral infection involves wide areas of mucous membrane and is only expressed when cooling and drying allow viral induction of papilloma formation. Venturi ventilation has been condemned by some as a possible means of disseminating papillomas in the tracheobronchial tree and lungs. This is only a theoretical consideration and does not stand the test of our clinical experience. In the past 15 years, the Otolaryngology department at Boston University has performed several thousand procedures on several hundred recurrent respiratory papilloma patients. The venturi ventilation system has been used frequently and repeatedly. Tracheobronchial or pulmonary dissemination has never been observed in any patient ventilated with a Venturi system who has not already had tracheobronchial involvement preceding use of the Venturi system. In these few cases the disease has obviously been a very aggressive form. The Venturi system actually aids in the precise vaporization of papillomas and appears to us to be without risk of associated dissemination.

In laryngeal disease recurring at varying intervals over many years, voice preservation is essential. As voice production requires only an adequate flow of air and perturbation of the air column, it is obvious that complete removal of papillomas is unnecessary. It is far better to leave a few small papillomas on the vocal folds than to risk vocal impairment.

A fundamental goal should be the avoidance of harm (Wetmore, Key and Suen, 1985). Overenthusiastic laser surgery producing denudation of the epithelial surface of the larynx inevitably produces problems. These include anterior and posterior webs, and extensive fibrosis and scarring which impairs vocal fold mobility and epithelial vibration. Not only is the voice compromised but severe stenosis can result. Such

The laser in laryngeal disease

overly enthusiastic therapy usually has no effect on the course of the disease.

(a) Treatment plan for recurrent respiratory papillomatosis (Simpson and Strong, 1983)

The first use of the CO_2 surgical laser in man was in the treatment of recurrent respiratory papillomatosis. This occurred in 1972 at Boston University Medical Center. Since that time the laser has proven its place as the treatment of choice in the surgical management of recurrent respiratory papillomatosis. The laser allows progressive vaporization of papillomas with excellent haemostasis. This permits a clear microscopic assessment of the disease and the effectiveness of surgery. A biopsy is taken with cup forceps. This may be the only direct manipulation of the papillomas required. Papillomas are gradually vaporized to the degree desired. The vaporization is continued to a level which is always at or above the mucous membrane. Care should be taken not to invade Reinke's space or muscle. Such invasion can produce fibrosis, scar formation and vocal impairment. When large volumes of papillomas must be vaporized the laser should be fired in repeated, 0.1 s bursts, or with rapid movement of the beam to avoid heat buildup in a local area. Continuous suction with a separate suction channel or a microsurgical suction tip is necessary to remove smoke and steam to ensure visibility and to prevent local heat injury.

All papillomas are removed from one cord and most of the other. Care is taken to spare 2 mm at the anterior end of the cord at the anterior commissure to prevent fibrotic web formation. When a few papillomas remain after the first surgery, the procedure is repeated in four weeks. If no recurrence in the treated area is seen at that time an attempt at cure is made by ablating all remaining lesions. This is an attempt to induce remission. If there is obvious regrowth in the treated areas therapy is thereafter limited to maintaining the airway and maximal voice quality while awaiting the later development of remission.

Papillomas occurring in a posterior vocal cord, the posterior commissure, or the posterior subglottic area are not readily vaporized with the endotracheal tube in place. In these situations the endotracheal tube is removed and ventilation is continued with the Venturi system.

3.9.9 KERATINIZING PAPILLOMA

The mucous membrane of the glottis normally does not produce keratin. The presence of keratin on a papilloma suggests the possibility of verrucous carcinoma. This requires a complete excisional biopsy

Specific benign organic lesions

including the base for careful histological examination by the pathologist. The entire lesion is excised *en bloc*. The mucosal cuts are outlined with the laser. The lesion is then grasped with cup forceps, placed under tension and then excised with the laser, with a 2 mm margin. Both keratinizing papillomas and verrucous carcinoma do not invade but rather push against nearby tissue as they increase in size. If the surgical margin is clear, no further treatment is necessary but periodic follow up is mandatory.

3.9.10 HYPERKERATOTIC PAPILLOMA

Hyperkeratotic papillomas are heaped up spikes of keratin over normal underlying connective tissue which is without the branching stalks seen in recurrent respiratory papillomatosis. Hyperkeratotic papillomas are not a true papilloma and the aetiology is unkown. Although these lesions are benign they may recur frequently after excision. All require excisional biopsy for histological examination for identification and to rule out malignancy which may have a quite similar appearance. The specimen is excised under tension after the mucosal cuts are outlined with the laser. An incision is made into Reinke's space, but care is taken to avoid the underlying muscle. The specimen is oriented and placed on a desiccated cucumber slide for serial sectioning and examination by the pathologist.

3.9.11 LARYNGOCOELE

A laryngocoele is a cystic enlargement of the laryngeal ventricle usually appearing within the glottis and displacing the false vocal fold into the lumen at the laryngeal inlet. These can become large enough to extend through the cricothyroid space to form an external laryngocoele which presents as a mass in the neck which enlarges during the modified valsalva manoeuvre. A surgeon should never forget that benign or malignant tumours of the glottis may actually precipitate laryngocoeles by obstructing the outlet of the ventricle. Therefore, all laryngocoeles require laryngoscopy and excision.

Laser surgical techniques allow endoscopic management of laryngocoeles. After exposing the internal laryngocoele with the Lynch suspension system or a wide bore (Jako-Kleinsasser) laryngoscope the surgeon opens the laryngocoele with the laser. This allows decompression with suction aspiration. The false vocal fold is then grasped with cup forceps and placed under tension by pulling it to the contralateral side. The laser is then used to cut through first the superior and then the inferior wall to amputate the false vocal cord, thereby marsupializing the sac.

The laser in laryngeal disease

Many external laryngocoeles have a wide mouth passage through the cricothyroid membrane leading from the internal to the external sac. Marsupialization of the internal larygocoele allows easy drainage of the external sac into the larynx. The laryngocoele is then no longer apparent or symptomatic. Preoperative dexamethasone (1 mg kg to a maximum of 20 mg) minimizes laryngeal oedema and tracheotomy is unnecessary. The patient can be discharged the day following surgery as he has no skin incisions and requires minimal analgesia. The patient is eating normally. It must be remembered that external laryngocoeles frequently may require open surgery for eradication.

3.9.12 HAEMANGIOMAS

Two types of haemangioma involve the larynx – capillary and cavernous – each requiring different management.

Capillary haemangiomas occur in infants and young children in the subglottic area usually posteriorly (an anterior midline swelling is more likely to be a congenital cyst). These haemangiomas may produce airway obstruction but do not affect the voice unless the vocal fold itself is involved.

Carbon dioxide laser vaporization is effective and relatively simple (Simpson et al., 1979; Healy et al., 1980). If obstruction is not severe, tracheotomy may be avoided. General anaesthesia is obtained with a small endotracheal tube or tracheotomy if present. Suspension laryngoscopy exposes the larynx. A small Dedo or ideally a Healy subglottic laryngoscope is essential for exposure. The endotracheal tube (if used) is withdrawn and ventilation continued with the Venturi system. After a biopsy is taken, vaporization with the laser commences. The laser is fired in shorts bursts (0.1 s) at 5–10 W. Conservative vaporization is employed only to the level of surrounding mucosa. Caution is necessary to avoid iatrogenic stenosis. The procedure may be repeated at a later time if necessary but usually one treatment suffices.

Cavernous haemangiomas occur in any age group in any area of the larynx. The CO_2 laser is not effective in these lesions as it cannot provide effective haemostasis and should rarely if ever be used. The Nd-YAG laser can be very effective because of its tissue penetration and beam scatter and the resultant deep coagulation (Gillis and Strong, 1983; Polanyi, 1983; Primrose et al., 1987).

A fibreoptic cable is necessary to deliver Nd-YAG laser energy to tissues. The fibre can be passed through a standard open-end laryngeal suction tip. This provides rigidity which aids in accurately directing the fibre to the desired point of application. Unless crystal contact tips are used, the fibre should *not* touch the tissue, as coagulated tissue adhering to the fibre tip will concentrate the energy there and destroy the

Specific benign organic lesions

fibre tip. The amount of energy delivered at the impact site is inversely proportional to the distance of the tip from the tissue. Because of tissue penetration and scatter of the Nd-YAG laser energy and potential significant tissue necrosis, this laser must always be fired in bursts of less than 0.5 s at no more than 40 W. Unlike the case with the CO_2 laser, tissue appearance immediately after Nd-YAG laser application is not a reliable predictor of later tissue necrosis (Gillis and Strong, 1983; Primrose et al., 1987). A very conservative and cautious approach is essential, even for experienced Nd-YAG laser surgeons.

The Nd-YAG laser energy is applied to the haemangioma at multiple sites. Blanching and some shrinkage is seen. The ultimate resulting necrosis is ten to twenty times that noted at the initial application.

Cryotherapy has been the treatment of choice for cavernous haemangiomas including those in the larynx. It will probably continue to have a role, even when more surgeons have gained experience with the Nd-YAG laser.

Both the Nd-YAG laser and cryosurgery produce marked reactive inflammatory oedema. For airway security, tracheotomy is absolutely essential when either modality is used together with preoperative dexamethasone.

3.9.13 LARYNGEAL STENOSIS (Figure 3.7)

Laryngeal stenosis may be congenital or acquired and is one of the most challenging problems in Laryngology. Both communication and the airway may be impaired. A variety of surgical techniques including both endoscopic and open surgical approaches may be helpful or may be met with failure. Laser procedures offer new approaches to these difficult problems.

(a) Supraglottic stenosis

Supraglottic stenosis may be of congenital or traumatic origin. If glottic and vocal fold function is intact, a part or all of the involved epiglottic and aryepiglottic folds and false vocal cord may be excised. Exposure requires Lynch Suspension or a wide-bore laryngoscope. Preoperative dexamethasone minimizes oedema. Postoperatively patients do well; aspiration is rarely evident and then is only temporary; the voice is unaffected.

(b) Glottic webs and synechiae

These may be congenital or traumatic in aetiology. All are opened relatively easily by cutting through them with the laser, knife or

The laser in laryngeal disease

scissors. These webs require no further treatment. A large raw surface will usually result in reformation of the web before epithelialization can occur. This can be prevented by endoscopic placement of a small keel cut from sialastic sheeting and secured with heavy nylon or stainless-steel suture passed percutaneously and secured over buttons and removed after 3–6 weeks. A temporary tracheostomy is usually necessary for patients with significant webbing. Posterior glottic stenosis with arytenoid fixation does not respond to endoscopic surgery. Its successful management requires open surgical correction.

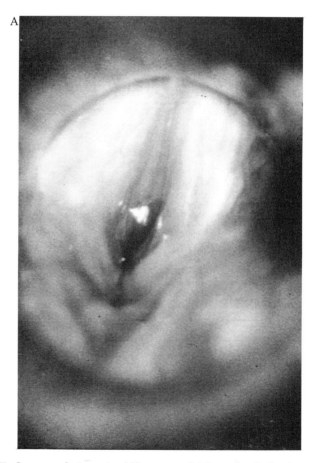

Figure 3.7 Laryngeal stenosis: (A) severe glottic and subglottic stenosis after intubation for croup, (B) stenosis excised and rolled silastic stent in position in larynx; (C) 6 months post-laser excision.

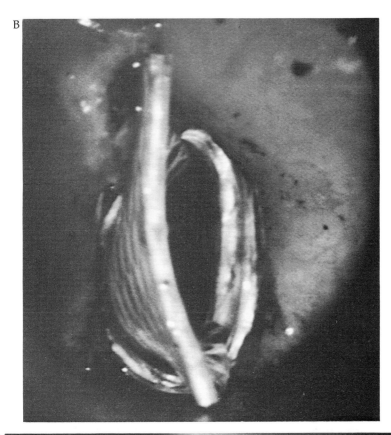
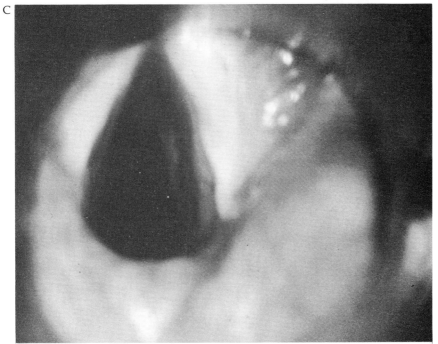

(c) Subglottic stenosis

Congenital laryngeal stenosis is the third commonest congenital laryngeal malformation (Holinger et al., 1976). It may be membranous or cartilaginous and is usually apparent in the first few weeks or months of life. Biphasic stridor and croup are the common presenting symptoms. Tracheotomy may be necessary before and during treatment (Holinger et al., 1976).

Acquired subglottic stenosis results from trauma. External blunt and penetrating forces, emergency high tracheotomy, caustic injuries and endotracheal intubation all may traumatize the larynx. New capabilities of advanced prolonged life support with prolonged and repeated endotracheal intubation have increased both the likelihood of traumatic laryngeal injuries and of acquired stenosis. Prolonged mechanical ventilation via an endotracheal tube produces direct pressure as well as shearing forces on laryngeal and tracheal mucosa with each inspiratory/expiratory cycle. Submucosal microvascular occlusion produces mucosal necrosis. Mucociliary flow is impaired. Infection frequently occurs and is a major factor in the resultant stenosis (Sasaki, Moriuchi and Koss, 1979; Simpson et al., 1982).

The stenosis may not be detected immediately. The patient is extubated and may seem to do well until an upper respiratory infection produces additional airway narrowing and respiratory distress. Fibrosis and scar contracture may progress and only become apparent after weeks or months.

A challenging problem, subglottic stenosis can be managed endoscopically or by open surgical (laryngofissure) methods. Treatment must be individualized and based on an accurate determination of the patient's problem and judicious selection of the treatment modality. Factors predicting failure of endoscopic management include circumferential scarring wider than 1 cm in vertical dimension, laryngomalacia from loss of cartilage, a history of severe bacterial infection complicating intubation, and posterior laryngeal inlet scarring with arytenoid fixation (Simpson et al., 1982). Initial endoscopic laser surgical management does not preclude open surgical techniques and may obviate the higher risk and longer hospitalization needed for open surgery.

Endoscopic management of stenosis includes endoscopic inspection, dilation for airway maintenance, and laser surgical correction (Friedman, Healy and McGill, 1983). Inspection is important in determining the extent of the problem and selecting the most appropriate treatment modality.

Gentle dilation helps to preserve the airway, while inflammatory oedema resolves and fibrosis matures, and (in children) the larynx and

Specific benign organic lesions

airway increase in size. It may be all that is necessary in mild stenosis but occasionally may prolong or increase stenosis especially if the surgeon is not gentle and further injury results. Dilation may maintain a lumen which will aid later endoscopic or open surgical management.

(d) Laser surgery for stenosis (Simpson et al., 1982; Friedman, Healy and McGill, 1983; Healy, 1982) (Figure 3.7)

Laser techniques offer several advantages. Surgical precision eliminates or minimizes damage to other tissues. Hospitalization is much shorter than that required for open surgical methods. Fewer procedures are required than for repeated dilatations. Tracheotomy is often avoided. If endoscopic laser surgery proves unsuccessful, open procedures can be performed without added risk.

In partial stenosis (less than 80% of crossectional area of normal lumen) several surgical sessions are necessary (Healy, 1982). Circumferential applications are avoided. Radial segments are vaporized with the laser. No stent is used. Prophylactic antibiotics minimize or prevent infection and further fibrosis.

In severe stenosis (greater than 80% lumen reduction), the entire area of fibrotic narrowing is excised (Healy, 1982). Soft silastic sheeting is fashioned in a roll as a stent in the larynx to maintain a lumen (Figure 3.7). The stent is secured with heavy nylon or wire suture tied over buttons on the skin. Antibiotics are necessary while the stent is in place. The stent is removed in four to six weeks.

While steroids have an anti-inflammatory effect and play an important role perioperatively to endoscopic procedures, they are not used postoperatively. Steroids impair epithelial migration and increase susceptibility to infection; both effects have been shown to increase scar formation and must be avoided.

Endoscopic laser management of stenosis is successful in carefully selected patients. Three to five procedures may be required. If success does not result, open methods usually will be required.

3.9.14 BILATERAL VOCAL CORD PARALYSIS–ARYTENOIDECTOMY

In cases of bilateral vocal cord abductor paralysis with airway compromise and occasionally in posterior glottic level stenosis or webbing with similar respiratory problems, endoscopic arytenoidectomy may prove beneficial and does not compromise or prevent the future use of other procedures. The goal is lateralization of one vocal fold to a degree producing an adequate glottic chink and airway, while recognizing the likely loss of vocal strength.

The laser in laryngeal disease

A temporary tracheotomy is necessary for airway security. With the patient under general anaesthesia, the surgeon places the larynx in suspension with an appropriate laryngoscope and then views the larynx with the operating microscope. Using the CO_2 laser, the surgeon exposes the arytenoid cartilage lateral to the vocal process and then dissects the cartilage free of all muscular attachments. Small arterial bleeding too brisk for laser haemostasis is controlled with the suction cautery or by clamping the artery with upbiting cup forceps and then firing the laser at the cup to heat-cauterize the vessel. Laryngeal microsurgical instruments including probes, scissors and hooks are necessary for disarticulation of the cricoarytenoid joint and extraction of the cartilage. A pyramidal shaped wedge of vocalis muscle (pointing anteriorly) is vaporized, while care is taken to preserve intact the mucosa of the free edge and subglottic surface of the vocal folds. The resultant cavity is obliterated by retracting the cord laterally with a heavy 2–0 or 3–0 nylon suture passed around the cord in the vocal process area. This suture is first passed through a 14 gauge needle passed percutaneously from the anterolateral skin of the neck into the laryngeal lumen in the subglottic area. The endolaryngeal end of the suture is pulled out through the laryngoscope. The needle is again passed percutaneously into the larynx above the vocal fold and the suture threaded from within the larynx into and through the needle which is then withdrawn. The nylon suture is tied over a button while assessing the degree of vocal fold lateralization with microlaryngoscopy. The lateralizing retention suture is retained for 2–3 weeks and then removed in the clinic. Prophylactic antibiotics are used during this period. Following removal of the retention suture, if the airway is satisfactory by indirect examination and airflow, the patient can be decannulated and the tracheotomy allowed to close. Occasionally as a result of infection or unusual inflammatory response, excessive fibrosis will occur. Correction requires laryngofissure for resection of fibrosis, mucosal transposition flaps and use of a soft silastic roll stent.

3.9.15 OTHER BENIGN PROBLEMS

Occasionally other rare problems such as neurofibromas, localized amyloid tumours, lymphangiomas, and other lesions may be managed endoscopically with the laser (Simpson *et al.*, 1979, 1984).

3.10 Premalignant and malignant disease

3.10.1 CARCINOGENESIS

Following repeated exposure to a number of substances, particularly tobacco products, epithelial tissue of the upper aerodigestive tract may

Premalignant and malignant disease

undergo gradual changes that culminate in invasive epidermoid carcinoma (Vaughan et al., 1980). This process may require many years. While cellular atypia may not be clinically apparent during this period, it can be detected by ultrastructural examination of affected mucosa and even on occasion by light microscopy (Incze et al., 1982). Mucosal abnormalities eventually develop which exhibit white or red patches variously termed cellular atypia, leukoplakia or carcinoma in situ (severe atypia). These conditions are considered premalignant while the basement membrane remains intact. There are only minor differences between these changes and all degrees of variation may be present in any particular lesion. Extension through the basement membrane represents invasive carcinoma rather than carcinoma in situ.

3.10.2 PREMALIGNANT DISEASE

(a) Keratosis

As the normal mucous membrane of the glottis has no keratin layer, the presence of any keratosis on the glottis is abnormal. Keratosis may develop in response to chronic trauma, similar to callus formation and is seen in long-standing vocal nodules. This common condition is not a premalignant condition. While keratosis without atypia is common, keratosis associated with atypia is premalignant. This condition may or may not present clinically as a white patch. The epithelial covering of the vocal folds may also appear dry, reddened, thickened, granular or roughened. The predominant histologic feature is epithelial atypia of varying degrees. Keratosis may be absent while the histological diagnosis is still 'leukoplakia'.

Papillary keratosis (hyperkeratotic papilloma) consists of white masses formed by spikes of keratin. These develop for unknown reasons. Histological examination reveals no atypia and flat underlying stroma with the branching stalks characterizing papillomas. Papillary keratosis produces vocal deterioration and a sensation of irritation.

(b) Carcinoma in situ (erythroplakia)

In carcinoma in situ, severe cellular atypia extends from the intact basement membrane of the epithelium to its surface. If the basement membrane is invaded, the lesion is invasive carcinoma. Carcinoma in situ has a reddish velvet appearance (erythroplasia) as there is no keratin on the surface and the lesion cannot appear white. Carcinoma in situ stains intensely with a supravital dye such as toluidine blue O.

Supravital staining is of great assistance in evaluating epithelial lesions as severe atypia and malignancy show intense staining (Strong

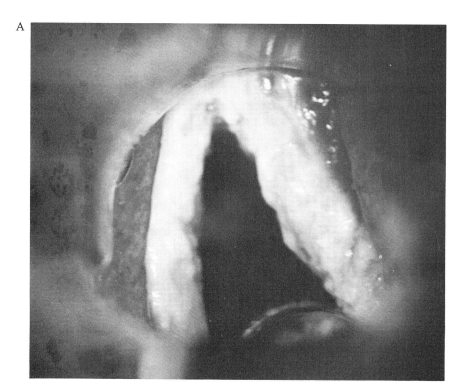
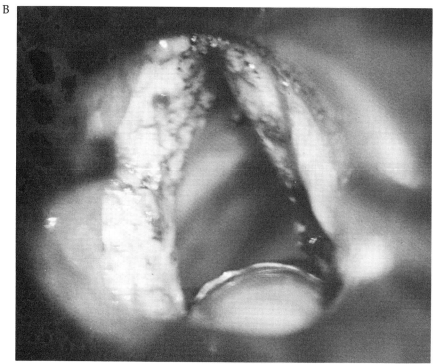

Premalignant and malignant disease

and Vaughan, 1970). Technique is important. Endoscopy and endotracheal intubation must be performed gently, preferably by more experienced individuals as minor traumatic lesions such as abraded mucosa will show increased staining and could confuse the clinical picture. The stain (toluidine blue O dye) is painted gently on the mucosa and then rinsed away after 20 s. A double-lumen laryngeal suction irrigation tip facilitates this cleansing. Normal mucosa remains unstained or only lightly stained while areas of atypia and malignancy show intense uptake of the dye which results in a dark blue to blue–black colour.

Excisional biopsy is the treatment for all keratotic (white) and erythroplastic (red) lesions (Blakeslee et al., 1983). This allows histological examination to rule out malignancy and also relieves symptoms (after healing). After induction of general endotracheal anaesthesia and complete muscle relaxation, the patient receives a complete endoscopic examination of the upper aerodigestive tract (laryngoscopy, oesophagoscopy and bronchoscopy) since multiple lesions are common. After placing an appropriate laryngoscope in suspension, the surgeon carefully examines the larynx with the operating microscope. The lesion is palpated with probes and stained with a supravital dye. Firing the CO_2 laser in bursts or continuously, the surgeon lightly incises the mucosa around the lesion, then grasps the lesion with cup forceps, gently applies tension, and excises the lesion with laser dissection in the plane of Reinke's space without violating the underlying muscle (unless obvious invasion is seen). The specimen is oriented and placed on a carrier substance such as desiccated cucumber. Small slices of cucumber can be stored in 95% alcohol for this purpose. The slice is allowed to dry and the biopsy specimen is laid flat on the slice for later histological examination. Egg white, fibrin glue, or a small amount of methylmethacrylate or 'Crazy Glue' can be used as an adhesive, but excessive amounts of plastic adhesive can damage microtome blades. Cutting a notch in one end of the cucumber slice helps orient the specimen which is then placed in formalin. Communication with the pathologist is essential as histological serial sectioning must be perpendicular to the surface, so as to allow an accurate determination of the extent and degree of atypia.

Figure 3.8 Vocal fold keratosis: (A) before excision; (B) immediately after excision in Reinke's space. Note that muscle is not exposed.

The laser in laryngeal disease

3.10.3 MALIGNANT DISEASE

In the management of laryngeal carcinoma, the CO_2 laser has proved to be a valuable instrument in several ways.

(a) Diagnosis

Whenever possible, excision biopsy (meticulous *en bloc* removal of the entire lesion (for histological examination of the complete and undistorted specimen) should be attempted. Most small lesions (premalignant and T_1 glottic carcinomas) are amenable to this technique. Panendoscopic examination of the upper aerodigestive tract is performed and all suspicious lesions are biopsied. With the operating microscope, the surgeon examines the larynx with suspension laryngoscopy, palpates the lesion and then stains it with toluidine blue O dye. With the CO_2 laser, the surgeon first outlines the lesion with a superficial mucosal incision, then grasps the lesion with cup forceps, applies tension, and excises the lesion in its entirety including vocalis muscle as necessary for complete removal. The specimen is oriented and then fixed to allow serial sectioning with cuts perpendicular to the surface. This specimen should be examined jointly by the surgeon and the pathologist to verify pertinent findings. The surgeon carefully evaluates the wound under 25× magnification. Inspection of the wound at this magnification allows identification of even a few abnormal cells which can be biopsied for frozen section examination as indicated. With this method of evaluation of the entire specimen, wound bed, and frozen section biopsies, the surgeon has an accurate diagnosis and knows the limits of the tumour. Repeat biopsies are unnecessary.

(b) Excision biopsy for cure (Figures 3.9–3.11)

These excision biopsy techniques can be curative if the entire tumour is removed. Blakeslee *et al*. (1984) reported the results in 103 cases of T_1 glottic carcinoma treated with excisional biopsy and resulting in 92% with at least a three year disease-free interval in 50 patients. These patients all met the following essential conditions: (1) the lesion was completely exposed at laryngoscopy, (2) the lesion did not involve the anterior commissure or vocal process, (3) the lesion was confined to the mucous membrane, (4) there was no further tumour visible on 25× magnification, (5) a frozen section biopsy specimen of the wound was free of disease, and (6) multiple permanent sections of the tumour showed disease-free margins. Six of 15 patients who had failed primary radiation elsewhere underwent excision biopsy which proved curative when the specimen margins were free of cancer.

Premalignant and malignant disease

While the laser is most beneficial and can be curative in localized, well-defined T_1 carcinoma, and especially verrucous carcinoma, higher staged tumours (T_2 and T_3) occasionally (rarely) can be excised if the sphincteric protective function is not thereby compromised. Such compromise results if both true and false vocal cords are excised on the same side. Such surgery should only be attempted by surgeons with a great deal of experience with endoscopic surgery.

Although it is desirable to have the excised specimen reveal margins which are free of tumour, it is not essential. At least 1–2 mm of margin are lost by laser vaporization of tissue during excision of the specimen. The only important excision margins are those of the wound bed. Careful examination of the wound under 25× magnification and appropriate frozen section biopsies of the wound bed are essential. If facilities for frozen section examination are not available, we would recommend that excision for cure is not attempted.

(c) Excision biopsy for staging

Staging is one of the most important benefits of use of the laser in laryngeal cancer. A subtotal excision of laryngeal tumours may allow a more exact determination of their true extent. Clinical staging based on indirect or direct examination may be inaccurate. T_1 glottic carcinoma by definition is confined to the vocal cord with both cords being mobile, implying that the tumour is confined to the surface epithelium without muscle invasion. We have found, however, that vocal fold mobility is an extremely inaccurate measurement of muscle invasion by tumour. At excision, many clinically staged T_1 tumours are found to invade muscle deeply and should be classified biologically and treated as T_3 tumours. A tumour 'T_1' at the anterior commissure with a mobile vocal fold may actually be a biologic T_4 lesion if it has broken through the thyroid cartilage. Using the laser, the tumour can be excised or gradually vaporized and followed until its true limits are determined.

Bulky supraglottic tumours may obscure their site of origin. Only after large amounts of tumour have been removed, can the surgeon determine whether the patient is a candidate for partial laryngeal (supraglottic) resection or will require total laryngectomy.

Using the laser for excision and dissection, the surgeon can perform more precise staging which in turn allows more accurate statistical evaluation of therapeutic results.

(d) Recurrent carcinoma after radiation therapy

Recurrent or residual carcinoma of the larynx after radiation therapy can be a difficult diagnostic problem. Cup forceps biopsies of surface

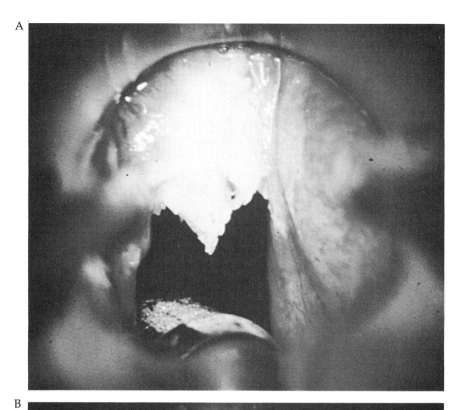

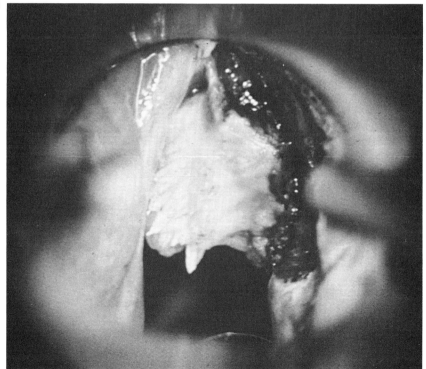

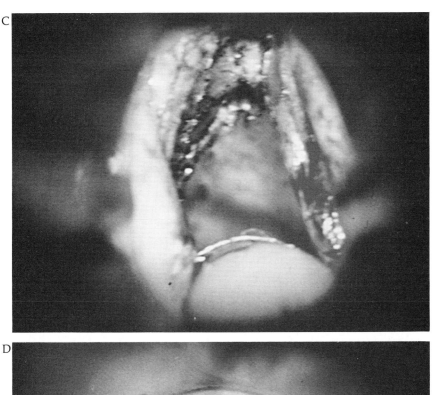

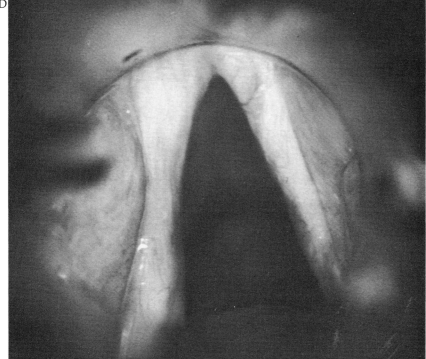

Figure 3.9 Verrucous carcinoma: (A) before excision; (B) partially excised; (C) completely excised; (D) one year after excision (no evidence of disease).

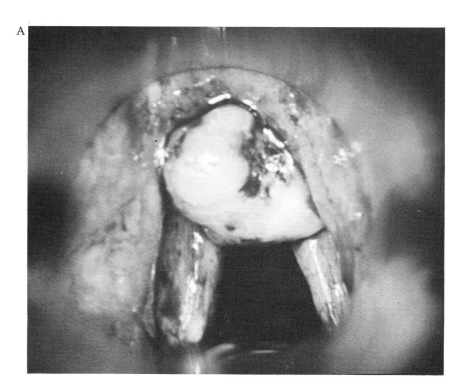

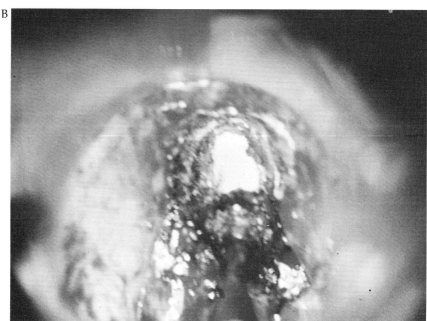

Premalignant and malignant disease

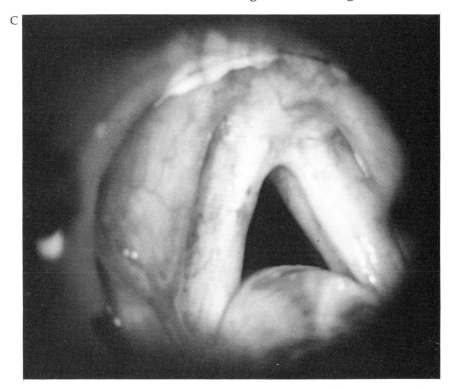

Figure 3.10 Sarcoma: (A) before excision; (B) excised; (C) two years after excision (no evidence of disease).

epithelium frequently are unrewarding until surface ulceration reveals the underlying carcinoma. The tumour may lie deep within the tissue and may be multicentric. Only serial sections of the vocal fold can reveal the disease. Using the CO_2 laser, the surgeon can excise the entire vocal fold anterior to the vocal process. The laser cut is made just anterior to the vocal process carried laterally to the thyroid cartilage and then forward along the perichondrium to the anterior commissure. The pathologist can then examine the entire vocal fold with serial sections to find residual carcinoma. If margins are clear of disease or no carcinoma is found, the patient is followed. The voice initially is very weak, but gradually improves as a result of compensatory movements of the opposite vocal fold and formation of a scar tissue pseudocord. The voice may show surprising improvement but usually shows residual hoarseness. Whereas obvious residual disease will mandate salvage surgery, some patients will be cured by excision biopsy (see above).

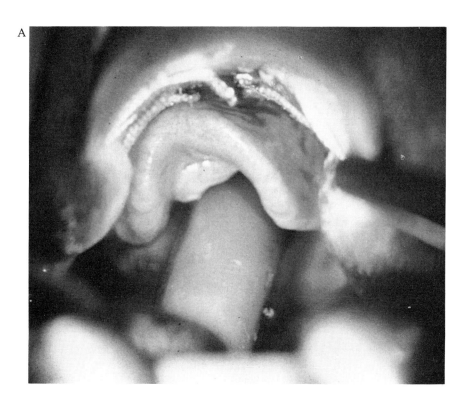

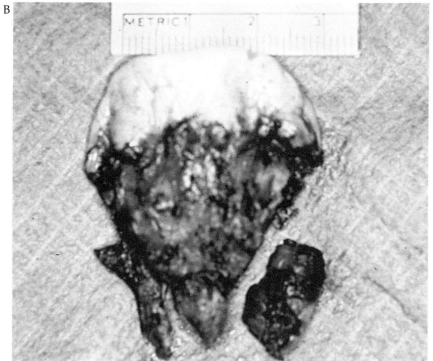

Premalignant and malignant disease

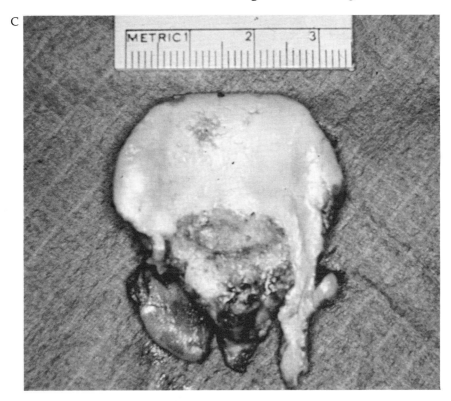

Figure 3.11 Epidermoid carcinoma of larynx: (A) excising epiglottis; (B) excised specimen (laryngeal surface – clear margins); (C) excised specimen (lingual surface – clear margins).

(e) Airway preservation

Bulky tumours obstructing the airway may be partially excised or vaporized with the laser to the extent required to re-establish an adequate airway. Tracheotomy can be avoided or postponed thereby eliminating many complications including wound sepsis, possible tracheal injury and possible peristomal seeding. Appropriate definitive therapy can then be selected and employed at lower risk.

(f) Cytoreduction ('Debulking')

While determining the extent of the tumour, the surgeon usually must excise or vaporize with the laser large amounts of tumour. This may be curative if the entire tumour is excised. Frequently only microscopic nests of tumour remain once the surgeon determines that endoscopic resection is not possible. In theory, the effectiveness of subsequent radiation therapy or chemotherapy should be enhanced since the tumour burden has been markedly reduced; but the long-term effects of cytoreduction as adjuvant therapy are unproven. If laryngeal sphincteric function is left intact cytoreduction produces little or no increase in morbidity. While the removal of large amounts of tumour may be tedious, the results are rewarding, as the general condition of the patient is often improved along with the airway and the abilities to eat, drink and communicate.

It is important to understand that endoscopic excision of even huge amounts of malignant tissue in no way interferes with future therapy. Postoperative morbidity is similar to that following simple endoscopic biopsy. With a secure diagnosis and accurate staging, the surgeon may select and promptly institute appropriate therapy, whether partial or total laryngectomy, radiotherapy or combined therapy. If the excision is curative, only careful follow up is necessary.

(g) *Current treatment plans for laryngeal malignancy* (Vaughan, Strong and Jako, 1978)

All patients must undergo a thorough evaluation including a complete history and physical examination, radiographs and laboratory studies including a search for metastases as indicated.

Patients receive a complete rigid endoscopic examination of the upper aerodigestive tract under general anaesthesia and muscle relaxation. Using the CO_2 laser, the surgeon performs excision biopsy if possible or tumour debulking if indicated. This allows accurate staging and cytoreduction.

Prior to definitive surgery or radiation therapy, if specimen margins are free of disease, excision biopsy may be curative. In cases of possible persistent or recurrent disease after radiation, the surgeon can use the laser to help obtain a large biopsy specimen for histological examination. This excision may be curative if margins are clear, but allows further surgery as necessary.

The advantages of this approach include accuracy and minimal morbidity. The limits of the tumour can be precisely determined while normal tissue is preserved. Patients experience minimal postoperative pain and undergo normal healing, require brief hospitalizations and are discharged one or two days after surgery with a useful voice and normal alimentation.

3.11 Summary

As a part of a comprehensive surgical system, laser surgical instruments provide exquisite precision in microscopic laryngeal surgery. In taking advantage of the benefits of laser techniques, the surgeon must both understand the complete surgical system as well as the laser itself. This system includes anaesthesia techniques, surgical instruments, surgical techniques to provide access and safety, and a logical approach to pathological problems. Effective use of the system requires careful patient selection and pre-operative and postoperative care. With careful attention to these details, the surgeon may realize unparalleled benefits in clinical efficacy while minimizing surgical complications, patient discomfort and the utilization of medical resources.

References

Andrews, A. H. Jr. and Baim, H. M. (1982), Accessor Instruments. In (eds A. H. Andrews, Jr and T. G. Polanyi, *Microscopic and Endoscopic Surgery with the CO_2 Laser* Littleton, John Wright, Bristol, pp. 111–21.

Blakeslee, D., Vaughan, C. W., Shapshay, S. M., Simpson, G. T., and Strong, M. S. (1983), Excisional biopsy in the selective management of keratosis, atypia, carcinoma in situ and microinvasive carcinoma of the larynx. *Am. J. Surg.*, **146**, 512–16.

Blakeslee, D., Vaughan, C. W., Shapshay, S. M., Simpson, G. T. and Strong, M. S. (1984), Excisional biopsy in the selective management of T_1 glottic cancer: A three year follow-up study. *Laryngoscope*, **94**, 488–94.

Costa, J., Howley, P. M., Bowling, M. C., Howard, R. and Baver, W. C. (1981), Presence of human papilloma viral antigens in juvenile multiple papilloma. *Am. J. Clin. Pathol.*, **75**, 194–7.

Davis, R. K. and Simpson, G. T. (1983), Safety with the carbon dioxide laser. *Otolaryngol. Clin. N. Am.*, **16**, 801–13.

Friedman, E. M., Healy, G. B. and McGill, T. J. (1983), Carbon dioxide laser management of subglottic and tracheal stenosis. *Otolaryngol. Clin. N. Am.*, **16**, 871–7.

Gillis, T. M. and Strong, M. S. (1983), Surgical laser and soft tissue interaction. *Otolaryngol. Clin. N. Am.*, **16**, 775–83.

Healy, G. B. (1983), Complications of laser surgery. *Otolaryngol. Clin. N. Am.*, **16**, 815–20.

Healy, G. B., Fearon, B. and French, R. *et al.* (1980), Treatment of subglottic hemangioma with the carbon dioxide laser. *Laryngoscope*, **90**, 809–13.

Healy, G. B. (1982), An experimental model for endoscopic correction of subglottic stenosis with clinical applications. *Laryngoscope*, **92**, 1103–15.

Holinger, P. H., Kutnick, S. N. and Schild, J. A. (1976), Subglottic stenosis in infants and children. *Ann. Otol. Rhinol. Laryngol.*, **85**, 591–9.

Incze, J. S., Vaughan, C. W., Lui, P. and Strong, M. S. (1982), Premalignant changes in normal appearing epithelium in patients with squamous cell carcinoma of the upper respiratory tract. *Am. J. Surg.*, **144**, 401–5.

Jackson, C. and Jackson, C. L. (1945), *Diseases of the Nose, Throat and Ear*. W. B. Saunders, Philadelphia, p. 433.

Lacina, O. (1972), Das Voukommen von Stimlippenknotchen bei den Sangern. *Folia Phoniat*, **24**, 345–54.

The laser in laryngeal disease

Lack, E., Jenson, A. B., Smith, H. G., Healey, G. B., Pass, F. and Vawter, G. F. (1980), Immuno-perioxidase location of papilloma virus in laryngeal papillomas. *Intervirology*, **14**, 148–54.

Norton, M. L. (1983), Anesthesia for laser surgery – laryngobronchoesophagology. *Otolaryngol. Clin. N. Am.*, **16**, 785–91.

Polanyi, T. G. (1983), Laser physics. *Otolaryngol. Clin. N. Am.*, **16**, 753–74.

Primrose, W., McDonald, G. A., O'Brien, M. T., Vaughan, C. W. and Strong, M. S. (1987), Synergistic effects of sequential carbon dioxide and Neodymium Yttrium Aluminum Garnet laser injuries: Experimental observations and measurements. *Ann. Otol. Rhinol. Laryngol.*, **96**, 47–52.

Sasaki, C. T., Moriuchi, M. and Koss, N. (1979), Tracheostomy related subglottic stenosis: bacteriologic pathogenesis. *Laryngoscope*, **89**, 857–65.

Simpson, G. T. and Strong, M. S. (1983), Recurrent respiratory papillomatosis: The role of the carbon dioxide laser. *Otolaryngol. Clin. N. Am.*, **16**, 887–94.

Simpson, G. T., Healy, G. B., McGill, T. and Strong, M. S. (1979), Benign tumors and lesions of the larynx in children: Surgical excision by CO_2 laser. *Ann. Otol. Rhinol. Laryngol.*, **88**, 479–85.

Simpson, G. T., Strong, M. S., Healy, G. B., Shapshay, S. M. and Vaughan, C. W. (1982), Predictive factors of success and failure in the endoscopic management of laryngeal and tracheal stenosis. *Ann. Otol. Rhinol. Laryngol.*, **91**, 384–8.

Simpson, G. T., Strong, M. S., Skinner, M. and Cohen, A. S. (1984), Localized amyloidosis in the head and neck and upper aerodigestive and lower respiratory tract. *Ann. Otol. Rhinol. Laryngol.*, **93**, 374–9.

Strauss, M. and Jenson, A. B. (1985), Human papillomavirus in various lesions of the head and neck. *Otolaryngol. Head Neck Surg.*, **93**, 343–6.

Strong, M. S. and Vaughan, C. W. (1970), Toluidine blue in the diagnosis of cancer of the larynx. *Arch. Otolaryngol.*, **91**, 515–19.

Strong, M. S., Vaughan, C. W., Mahler, D. G., Jaffe, D. R. and Sullivan, R. C. (1974), Cardiac complications of microsurgery of the larynx. Etiology, Incidence and Prevention. *Laryngoscope*, **84**, 908–20.

Strong, M. S., Vaughan, C. W., Cooperband, S. R. and Clement, M. A. C. P. (1976), Recurrent respiratory papillomatosis: Management with the CO_2 laser. *Ann. Otol. Rhinol. Laryngol.*, **85**, 508–16.

Vaughan, C. W., Strong, M. S. and Jako, G. J. (1978), Laryngeal carcinoma: Transoral treatment utilizing the CO_2 laser. *Am. J. Surg.*, **136**, 490–3.

Vaughan, C. W., Homburger, F., Shapshay, S. M., Soto, E. and Bernfield, P. (1980), Carcinogenesis of the upper aerodigestive tract. *Otolaryngol. Clin. N. Am.*, **13**, 405–12.

Wetmore, S. J., Key, J. M., Suen, J. Y. (1985), Complications of laser surgery for laryngeal papillomatosis. *Laryngoscope*, **95**, 798–801.

4 Endoscopic laser surgery of the tracheobronchial tree
Role of the CO_2 and Nd-YAG Lasers

GRAEME A. MCDONALD AND M. STUART STRONG

The passage of laser beams through rigid or flexible bronchoscopes has added an exciting new dimension to the diagnosis and treatment of airway disease. The initial clinical report of laser bronchoscopy by Strong et al. (1974) described 15 cases treated with the CO_2 laser through a rigid bronchoscopic system. Since then its use has expanded to allow the removal of benign lesions as well as palliation of malignant diseases obstructing the trachea and bronchi. More recently, the introduction of the Neodymium Yttrium, Aluminum, Garnet (Nd-YAG) laser through the flexible bronchoscope has permitted improved photocoagulation of vascular lesions of the tracheobronchial tree (Shapshay, Beamis and Dumon, 1985).

4.1 The CO_2 laser system

Until 1974 the CO_2 endoscopic delivery system consisted of a laser reflecting unit housed in a cubical box measuring 15 cm^3 to which the delivery tube was attached. This unit was fitted to a 3.5 mm × 30 cm or a 5 mm × 30 cm standard Jackson–Pilling bronchoscope. This original system was large, heavy and awkward to use (Figure 4.1).

In 1974, the endoscopic delivery system was made smaller, lighter and easier to handle and was coupled more conveniently to the bronchoscope. The CO_2 laser beam was directed down the bronchoscope by a highly reflective mirror and focused at its distal end by a lens. A dichroic mirror or beam splitter that is fully transmissive to the 10.6 μm laser radiation and fully reflective for visible light, allowed the operative site to be seen through an offset eye piece. The laser beam was aimed by adjusting two thumb screws which positioned the beam in the bronchoscope lumen. The beam spot size was approximately 2 mm in diameter, producing rather low power densities (Figure 4.2).

More recently, the delivery system has been further scaled down and

Endoscopic laser surgery

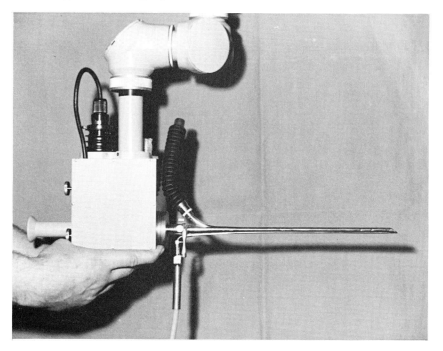

Figure 4.1 Original CO_2 endoscopic delivery system was too large and heavy for easy use.

made considerably more convenient to handle (Figure 4.3). The dichroic mirror was changed to a coated quartz crystal that is fully reflective to 10.6 μm wave length and transmissive to visible light. Although there is a minor offsetting of the eye piece with a refractive transparent plastic lens to allow for the linkage of a joystick, the optics have been improved along with improved control of the bronchoscope and laser beam. A visible helium neon aiming beam accurately predicts the site of impact of the invisible CO_2 beam.

Anaesthesia is induced with theopentothal and succinyl choline permitting the introduction of the bronchoscope. If the patient has a pre-existing tracheotomy or endotracheal tube, the patient is extubated as the bronchoscope is introduced transorally. When the airway has been established with the bronchoscope, anaesthesia is maintained by inhalation of non-flammable anaesthetic gases through the ventilating side port of the bronchoscope using not less than 90% O_2 concentrations (Figure 4.4).

An inflatable rubber cuff is used at the distal aspect of the bronchoscope to obtain better ventilatory control and permit positive pressure

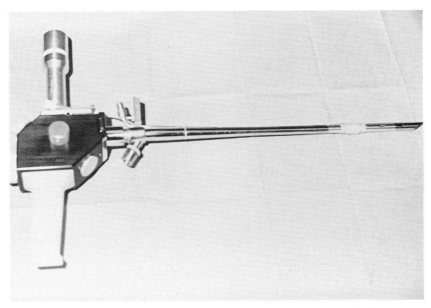

Figure 4.2 Improved housing of the endoscopic coupler made the laser coupling to the bronchoscope easier and more convenient to handle.

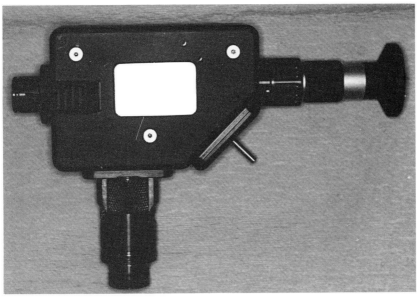

Figure 4.3 The most recent CO_2 laser coupler is extremely light and easy to handle, with a single joystick and clip-on coupler.

Endoscopic laser surgery

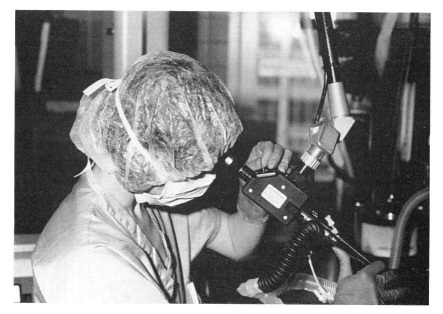

Figure 4.4 Laser bronchoscopy is shown in use with the patient under general anaesthesia maintained by inhalation anaesthesia through the side port of the bronchoscope.

breathing. Bronchoscopes used for laser surgery are designed without distal ventilation ports on the side in order to prevent accidental ignition of the rubber cuff where it may cover the existing port. Where there are existing ventilation ports on the bronchoscopes, they may be adapted for laser surgery by covering the ports with 1 cm self-adhering metallic aluminum tape. The rubber cuff may be placed over this protective covering. The balloon of the cuff is filled with water as an added protection against accidental ignition from air-borne incendiary particles (Figure 4.5).

The bronchoscope may be advanced as needed into the trachea or bronchi to evaluate the extent of the disease. The Hopkins Rod Telescope may be inserted through the rigid bronchoscope to give a magnified and more brightly illuminated view of the area to be treated (Figure 4.6). With the CO_2 system, the telescope must be removed before attaching the laser endoscopic coupler to the bronchoscope in preparation to systematically vaporizing the lesion. When the airway has been significantly reduced by the lesion in the tracheobronchial tree, the bronchoscope must be carefully advanced beyond the obstruc-

The CO_2 laser system

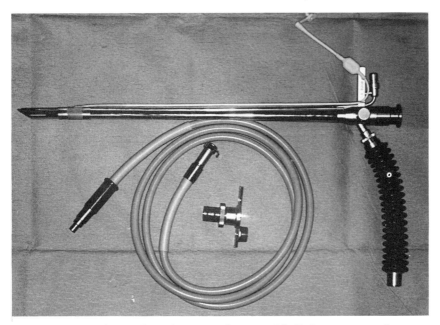

Figure 4.5 Ventilating bronchoscope shown with light source and water-inflatable rubber cuff.

tion to insure adequate ventilation. Vaporization may then begin at the most distal area and proceed to the proximal aspect of the obstruction. Vaporization of the lesion is continued until the tracheal or bronchial walls are free of gross disease (Figures 4.7 and 4.8). Despite care being taken to minimize bleeding secondary to manipulation of the bronchoscope, tumours are often friable and vascular and bleeding may obscure the normal anatomical landmarks of the distal airway; destruction of the lesion is often slow and tedious. The tidal flow of ventilatory gases consisting of halothane and more than 90% O_2 through the bronchoscope helps to maintain the field free of steam and smoke. On occasion, brisk bleeding may be encountered and haemostasis can be re-established by tamponading with topical 1/10 000 epinepherine, or electrocoagulation with an insulated suction tube.

When the laser excision is complete, anaesthesia is terminated and the bronchoscope is withdrawn. The patient is reintubated with an endotracheal tube and allowed to wake up permitting suctioning of secretions. In most cases, extubation is accomplished in the OR or Recovery Room.

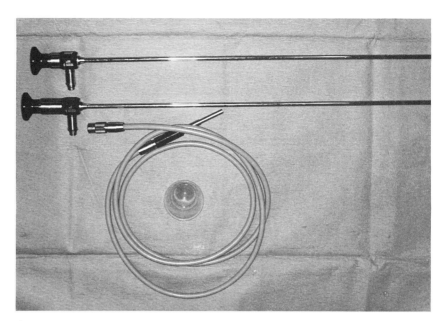

Figure 4.6 Hopkin Rod Telescopes with 0° and 90° lens give a magnified and better illuminated view of the airway.

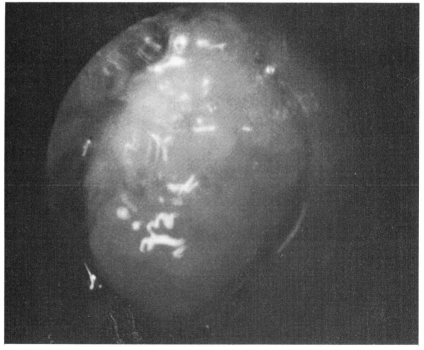

Figure 4.7 Osteochondroma shown obstructing right bronchus.

Nd-YAG laser system

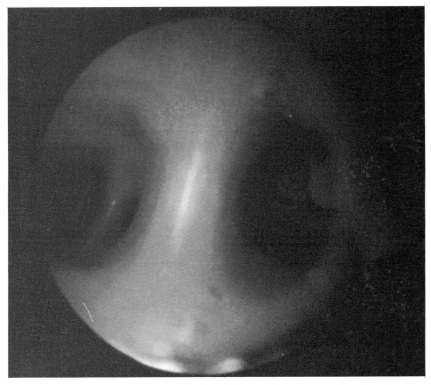

Figure 4.8 Postoperative view of the airway shown months after tumour removal.

4.2 Nd-YAG laser system

The Nd-YAG laser has been used increasingly in the treatment of tracheobronchial disease since the early 1980s. The 1.06 μm wavelength has markedly different properties from that of the CO_2 laser from the point of view of its soft tissue interaction and its delivery system. The YAG laser may be delivered through a flexible quartz fibre. This allows the laser energy to be carried directly to the lesion through the fibre in a flexible bronchoscope or through the side port of a rigid bronchoscopic system. With a white aiming light, the fibre may be directed onto or around the lesion. In either the rigid or flexible systems, the proximal optics used with the CO_2 system are replaced by a visually superior, magnified distal optical system. With the rigid bronchoscope the Hopkins Rod Telescope may be used to visualize tissue destruction as the Nd-YAG laser is being used.

Endoscopic laser surgery

Ventilation and anaesthesia are provided in a similar fashion; however, a suction catheter may be used through a second side port in the Dumon bronchoscope to aspirate smoke, blood and small particulate matter.

4.3 Soft tissue interaction

The soft tissue interaction of these lasers is due mainly to two materials found in biological tissues; water and haemoglobin. Haemoglobin has a high absorption for visible light of a short wavelength. Conversely, water has a high absorption for longer wavelengths in the infrared spectrum. The CO_2 laser with a 10.6 μm wavelength has a high absorption in water whereas the Nd-YAG has high absorption in haemoglobin and to a minimal extent in water.

All lasers used in surgery are in the visible or infrared region of the electromagnetic spectrum and their interaction with soft tissues leads to heating. The CO_2 and Nd-YAG wavelength are in the infrared region. Both lasers work through a process of tissue coagulation and/or vaporization secondary to heating. The nature and extent of the surgical wound depends upon the wavelength of the radiation, the absorption of the radiation, the intensity of the radiation and the total energy delivered to the tissues. The radiation of the CO_2 wavelength and that of the Nd-YAG laser interact very differently with tissues. On the one hand, the CO_2 wavelength is instantly absorbed and dissipated by as little as 0.03 mm of water; in biological tissues the effect is similar and there is no significant reflection or scattering of the energy. On the other hand the Nd-YAG wavelength is transmitted freely through water (up to 60 mm) but is strongly absorbed by red or black targets (haemoglobin or carbon particles); in biological tissue one-third of the energy is absorbed, one-third is transmitted and one-third is reflected with back scattering.

The differences between the CO_2 and Nd-YAG laser interactions with soft tissue are well demonstrated in the surgical setting. The CO_2 laser is a pure cutting beam which will coagulate vessels less than 0.5 mm. Its impact leaves a discrete crater with minimal tissue charring coagulation and oedema. It is a true laser scapel. The Nd-YAG laser, however, is primarily a coagulator of tissue but may vaporize tissue if surface charring develops. Since pigmentation may vary in soft tissue depending upon its vascularity, soft tissue interaction with the Nd-YAG laser is unpredictable and careful limitation of the power output and the time exposure is necessary to produce a therapeutic result safely. Its impact on soft tissue initially causes a circular area of blanched, denatured tissue. It will form a crater depending upon power density and the presence of surface charring. Sometimes a popcorn effect is seen where the epithelial layer elevates and bursts open forming a crater. Unlike the CO_2 laser, the Nd-YAG laser will cause surrounding tissue oedema and coagulation around the crater. As there is a variable degree of penetration with the Nd-YAG laser, there is ongoing necrosis of surrounding tissue over a period of one week. This results in expansion of the initial lesion, increased inflammatory response, and delayed wound healing. There is increased scarring. The Nd-YAG laser is not a pure cutting instrument but with its capacity to photo-coagulate vessels up to 4 mm, vascular lesions such as haemangiomas can be photo-coagulated with the YAG laser followed by ablation either with the YAG or CO_2 laser systems.

4.4 Indications

The indications for endoscopic use of a laser are relief of intrinsic tracheobronchial obstruction and control of tracheobronchial bleeding. The laser is useful during bronchoscopy to control haemorrhage following a punch biopsy. Coagulation of the site may be done with the Nd-YAG laser or, for small vessels, with a defocused beam of the CO_2 laser. Continuous suction down a separate port may be necessary to ensure a clear visual field during laser application.

Intrinsic airway obstruction secondary to benign lesions is the major indication for laser surgery. Recurrent respiratory papillomatosis is the most common lesion. In most cases these patients present with laryngeal papillomatosis and associated seeding into the trachea and bronchi. Of patients requiring tracheostomy for relief of laryngeal obstruction, 75% subsequently develop tracheobronchial papillomas. Laser destruction of the papillomas relieves the airway obstruction but repeated laser surgery is usually necessary to maintain the airway and allow subsequent extubation. While laser surgery may eradicate all visible papillomas in the tracheobronchial tree, long-term remission may occur spontaneously at any time but late recurrences are common.

Several endotracheal or bronchial lesions including amyloidosis, sarcoidosis, peristomal granulation and chondromas, etc. are amenable to laser destruction.

Tracheobronchial amyloid deposits bleed even with the most gentle manipulation and lend themselves to laser ablation. Since the amyloid may have destroyed the cartilaginous rings of the trachea, great care must be exercised if tracheal perforation is to be avoided. Only the redundant obstructing masses of amyloid should be destroyed.

Endoscopic laser surgery

Tracheal stenosis with tracheomalacia, may be ablated if the stenosis is web-like or less than 1 cm in length. Cicatrical stenoses involving a length of greater than 1 cm require open procedures with sleeve resection and end-to-end anastomosis of the trachea.

Many malignant tumours of the tracheobronchial tree present with airway obstruction; because of the degree of obstruction or associated sepsis, it may not be possible to initiate standard surgical or radiotherapeutic treatment. In most cases the airway can be restored temporarily using either or both the CO_2 and Nd-YAG laser endoscopically; thereafter appropriate resection or radiotherapy can be carried out promptly. Vascular tumours such as carcinoid will respond to Nd-YAG coagulation; thereafter the lesions can be vaporized with the CO_2 laser. Palliation of intrinsic obstruction in patients who have failed standard therapy with surgery and/or radiotherapy may or may not be indicated and must be evaluated on an individual basis. Recurrent tumours such as adenoidcystic carcinoma are particularly suitable for endoscopic destruction because they recur so slowly and may require only one laser excision per year for many years. Other forms of cancer, such as squamous cell, recur so rapidly (in two to three weeks) that one wonders if the intervention is worthwhile.

4.5 Contraindications

Extrinsic compression of the tracheobronchial airway by mass lesions is an absolute contraindication to laser surgery and tracheal stenosis due to tracheomalacia is unsuitable for laser resection. Since the CO_2 and Nd-YAG lasers must be applied to a relatively dry field, brisk active haemorrhage cannot be effectively coagulated by a laser unless the field can be kept clear by suctioning so that photo-coagulation can proceed with the Nd-YAG laser.

4.6 Pre-operative and postoperative evaluation

All patients being evaluated for laser bronchoscopy require the routine admission workup involved in any major surgical procedure. Blood analysis including complete blood count, platelet count, coagulation studies including PT and PTT, serum electrolytes and arterial blood gas levels are carried out. Chest X-rays are routinely done; when possible objective evaluation of the patient's airway is assessed pre-operatively by pulmonary function tests and tomography. Virtually all patients will have already undergone flexible fibreoptic bronchoscopy under local

Complications

anaesthetic, in order to assess the presence or absence of extrinsic compression and to determine the feasibility of laser surgery. Patients should be cross matched for blood as exsanguinating haemorrhages, although infrequent, may occur.

Postoperatively the patient is carefully monitored with arterial blood gases and serial chest X-rays. Length of stay in hospital is variable depending upon the severity of obstruction and whether there are any postoperative complications. Most patients are discharged within several days after their endoscopy.

4.7 Complications

With the employment of safety precautions the incidence of complication with laser bronchoscopic surgery is low; however, when they do occur the morbidity and mortality are high.

Brisk haemorrhage is more commonly seen with malignant airway disease or in cases where there have been numerous endoscopic procedures for amyloidosis or papillomas, etc. In these cases, erosion into a bronchial artery may occur due to tumour invasion or due to a weakening of the bronchial wall from repeated laser endoscopic procedures. These cases are generally not amenable to external control of the haemorrhage through a thoracotomy and the bleeding may have to be controlled by endobronchial packing with epinepherine and thrombin-soaked gauze for 24–48 h.

Ignition of the inflatable rubber cuff which is fitted over the bronchoscope near the distal end for better ventilation cannot occur if the ventilating ports of the bronchoscope have been closed with metallic tape or the laser bronchoscope is devoid of side ports.

Dislodged tumour fragments may travel distally causing temporary obstruction of one or both bronchi; these fragments and blood clots, etc. must be removed with suction and irrigation.

Tracheobronchial wall perforations may occur in cases where the cartilaginous wall has been destroyed by tumour or other disease, unless resection is confined to the obstructive mass only. It is always more prudent to under treat than over treat because tracheobronchial perforation may well prove to be fatal.

Cardiac arrhythmias leading to postoperative myocardial infarction are a serious threat. Because of the intensity of the airway manipulation and the frequent presence of multiple cardiac risk factors in these patients, any arrhythmias must be dealt with promptly and if possible the procedure terminated. Maintenance of high oxygen flow rates with greater than 90% concentration will reduce myocardial irritability and

Endoscopic laser surgery

reduce the build up of threatening levels of carbon monoxide in protracted procedures.

Postoperative atelectasis may occur but can usually be dealt with without any long-term sequelae.

4.8 Discussion

When compared to other endoscopic treatment with methods such as electrocoagulation, cryosurgery and radon seed application, laser bronchoscopic surgery has the advantage of localized soft tissue effect, less postoperative oedema, and a 'no touch' technique avoiding tumour manipulation and decreasing the possibility of haemorrhage. The effects of other methods of therapy are much less predictable. Laser surgery may be repeated whenever necessary, since there is no ionizing radiation and healing is prompt and complete after each application.

The CO_2 laser's main advantage is that it is a precise 'cutting' instrument and the soft tissue reaction in the normal tissue at the margin of the incision shows only 100 μm of cellular necrosis. There is essentially no postoperative oedema of the surrounding tissue and wound healing is rapid with little scar tissue formation. Its main disadvantage is that delivery is required through a rigid bronchoscopic system which makes access to the segmental bronchi impossible. The proximal optical system used in the CO_2 endoscopic coupler is poor, although the Hopkins Rod Telescope may be used to view the target area and monitor the progress of the operation intermittently. Although the CO_2 laser coagulates vessels less than 0.5 mm in diameter, it will not photocoagulate larger vessels feeding the tumour or vascular lakes.

The Nd-YAG laser complements the CO_2 laser in endoscopic surgery. Since it is efficiently conducted through a quartz fibre, the Nd-YAG laser may be used through a flexible bronchoscopic system enabling treatment of lesions at the orifices of the secondary bronchi. Through the rigid bronchoscopic system a Hopkins Rod Telescope can be introduced alongside the flexible quartz fibre providing an unsurpassed view of the lesion to be coagulated. The Nd-YAG laser is effective in coagulating vascular lesions such as angiomas or carcinoid tumours, etc.; thereafter the Nd-YAG laser can be used to vaporize the coagulated tissue if some carbonization has developed or the CO_2 laser can be used instead.

The use of the Nd-YAG laser through the flexible fibrescope, however, is limited to patients without any rigid obstruction in whom bleeding is not anticipated. Usually the rigid bronchoscopic system is preferred so that the airway can be secured and bleeding, if any, managed.

The Nd-YAG laser is not a pure cutting instrument such as the CO_2 laser; beyond the visible area of tissue destruction or coagulation, tissue changes occur which will result in delayed necrosis during the following four to five days. This effect, of course, is sometimes desirable. By limiting the use of the Nd-YAG laser to short intervals of 0.5–1.0 s and the power to 50 W more predictable responses are seen and the risk of extensive delayed tissue necrosis is minimized. More recently a sapphire tip has been applied to the flexible fibre which enables the focusing of the Nd-YAG laser energy to a fine point with high power density. Although the laser wavelength is the same, the high power density enables the instrument to vaporize tissue while limiting the depth of tissue penetration and scatter. The laser energy is applied by direct contact of the sapphire tip to the tissue. Experience in the tracheobronchial tree is limited with this form of delivery, however; it holds promise for the future.

Dye lasers and the use of haematoporphin derivatives continue to be investigated but at the present time they seem to be only of value in the diagnosis and treatment of carcinoma in situ or early bronchial tumours.

4.9 Summary

Endoscopic application of CO_2 and Nd-YAG lasers is a valuable method of treatment of selected tracheobronchial lesions causing obstruction. In some cases it may be the treatment of choice for benign airway disease, e.g. papillomatosis or amyloidosis. In obstructive malignant lesions of the tracheobronchial tree, laser surgery is valuable when definitive treatments (i.e. surgery, radiotherapy and chemotherapy) cannot be instituted or have failed. Patients selected for endoscopic laser surgery must be carefully evaluated and caution used to minimize morbidity and mortality. Although there continue to be rapid advances and refinements in laser technology, endoscopic laser surgery can be considered to be the standard treatment in selected cases.

References

Shapshay, S. M., Dumon, J. F. and Beamis, J. B. (1985), Endoscopic treatment of tracheobronchial tumors – experience with YAG and CO_2 lasers (506 operations). *Otolaryngol. Head Neck Surg.*, **93**, 205–10.

Strong, M. S., Vaughan, C. W., Polanyi, T. and Wallace, R. (1974), Bronchoscopic carbon dioxide laser surgery. *Ann. Otol. Rhinol. Laryngol.*, **83**, 769–76, 1974.

5 CO_2 laser surgery in the oral cavity

P. H. RHYS EVANS and J. W. FRAME

The recent introduction of the CO_2 laser has provided surgeons with a versatile tool which has proved most valuable in the treatment of many soft tissue lesions in the oral cavity. Because of the unique manner in which it interacts with and destroys living tissue the laser has introduced a new dimension in therapy combining many of the advantages of conventional surgical techniques. Not only does it offer a versatile method of excising or ablating tissue, but the healing process following therapy differs in many respects from that following conventional surgical excision. In the mouth where preservation of function and mobility following tissue excision is of prime importance, the reduction in contraction and scarring following laser therapy is an additional advantage.

5.1 Alternative surgical techniques: uses and limitations

Until the advent of the CO_2 laser, existing methods of excising or ablating tissue in the oral cavity included sharp dissection, the cutting diathermy and the cryoprobe. Each technique has its own merits and disadvantages which influence its use in particular situations, in addition to personal preferences and availability.

Excessive bleeding may be a problem with sharp dissection especially in such a vascular area as the mouth. This may hinder accurate excision, particularly of large superficial patches of leukoplakia where unnecessary removal of the underlying muscle layer will promote scar contracture.

Bleeding is reduced with the cutting diathermy which makes this technique more suitable for excision of tumours and deeper lesions. However, thermal damage caused by heat conduction away from the line of excision makes this instrument quite unsuitable for treatment of superficial patches of leukoplakia because these lesions need to be preserved for accurate histological evaluation. The linear burn from cutting diathermy will also cause extensive cell damage to adjacent tissue and the resulting inflammatory response may produce considerable postoperative oedema and pain.

The third possible method is the cryoprobe which may be used for ablation of superficial lesions and also in palliation of large ulcerating tumours. Its use is restricted by several disadvantages including inaccurate and unpredictable margins of destruction, the absence of a histological specimen and marked postoperative oedema with unpleasant slough formation.

5.2 The CO_2 laser: advantages

The CO_2 laser is a versatile instrument which combines many of the attributes of the other techniques both as a 'bloodless scalpel' and as a method of destroying tissue. These advantages are described in detail elsewhere but include precise dissection of tissue with instantaneous tissue vaporization. The sealing of blood vessels and lymphatics less than 0.5 mm in diameter allows relatively bloodless dissection and limits use of ligatures to larger vessels. Dissection can be carried out either with the handpiece (Figure 5.1) or under magnified control using the 'joystick' and laser attachment on the operating microscope (Figure 5.2). Improved access is achieved with the laser particularly for treatment of posterior lesions because of minimal instrumentation that is required. Under normal circumstances only retractors and suction are required. Accurate excision also allows preservation of the lesion for histological examination.

Damage to adjacent tissue is limited to a few cells and during the immediate postoperative period the inflammatory reaction, oedema and pain are minimal. This allows many intraoral resections to be safely carried out without the precaution of a temporary tracheostomy which inevitably would prolong the patient's stay in hospital. In the longer term, healing following laser therapy results in less contracture and scarring so that in many instances skin grafts and pedicled flaps are not required to fill the excised defect.

5.3 Use of the CO_2 laser in the mouth

Increasing experience with the CO_2 laser in surgery of the oral cavity has shown that in order to maximize the advantages of the instrument, several factors should be considered by the surgeon prior to treatment,

Use of the CO_2 laser in the mouth

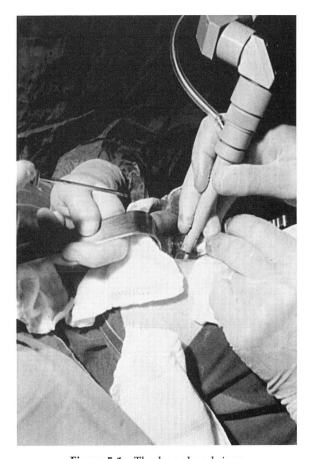

Figure 5.1 The laser handpiece.

especially where there is a choice between the handpiece and the operating microscope. Unlike the scalpel and diathermy, the physical properties of the laser beam can be varied considerably to suit dissection of different types of lesion in the mouth. The first group of factors relate to the laser beam itself and the second to the mucosal lesion being treated.

5.3.1 LASER VARIABLES

The penetration of the laser beam into the tissue surface can be modified by altering the spot size, the power density and the duration of exposure.

CO_2 laser surgery in the oral cavity

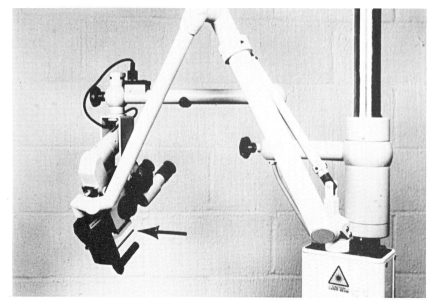

Figure 5.2 The laser attached to the operating microscope (arrow indicates 'joy-stick' control).

(a) Spot size

The spot size depends on the focal length of the converging lens through which the laser beam passes, either in the handpiece (125 mm) or on the operating microscope (300–400 mm). A shorter focal length produces a much finer spot and with the handpiece a small spot size of 0.2 mm can be achieved which is ideal for fine dissection. The beam can be rapidly defocused by withdrawing the handpiece from the surface a few more millimetres when coagulation of small vessels is required. When the microscope is used with the laser in the mouth a 300 mm lens is the optimum length because this allows the instrument to be sufficiently far away from the tissue surface for unimpeded use of retractors and yet it gives a fairly small spot size (0.6 mm). The 200 mm lens focuses to a smaller spot size (0.45 mm) but the microscope is too near the surface to allow adequate room for instrumentation.

Although a small spot achieved with the handpiece is preferable for fine dissection and deep biopsy excisions, the larger spot is ideal for surface vaporization because this treats the area more rapidly. Also the magnified image and the precise joystick control using the operating microscope makes this more suitable for accurate removal of large surface areas of leukoplakia.

Use of the CO_2 laser in the mouth

Table 5.1 Spot size and lens combinations

	Laser lens (mm)	Optical lens (mm)	Spot size (mm)
Handpiece	125	–	0.22
Microscope	200	200	0.45
	300	300	0.6
	400	400	0.8

Table 5.1 summarizes the different spot sizes achieved with different lens combinations using the handpiece or operating microscope. For dissection in the posterior part of the tongue and in the pharynx, the microlaryngoscope with 400 mm lenses is essential because of the extra distance involved. In these situations the spot size of 0.8 mm is adequate for most dissections and for obtaining biopsy material.

(b) Power density

The power density is the effective penetrating power of the laser beam at the tissue surface. This depends on the size of the spot and the power setting on the laser console. Table 5.2 shows the wide variation in power density achieved with different spot sizes, ranging from 105 290 W/cm^2 using the handpiece to 7968 W/cm^2 using the 400 mm lens, both at the 40 W power setting on the console.

In practical terms this variation in power is of importance to the surgeon when choosing an appropriate method of excision for a given procedure. Where a large tongue tumour is being resected using the laser as a knife, the powerful narrow beam obtained with the handpiece is ideal. At a power setting of 30 W the power density achieved is almost 80 000 W/cm^2 (Table 5.2). Excising the same lesion with the operating microscope and 300 mm lens at the same power setting of

Table 5.2 Power density and lens combination (W/cm^2)

	Lenses	Spot size (mm)	10 W	20 W	30 W
Handpiece	125/–	0.22	26 322	52 645	78 968
Microscope	200/200	0.45	6 291	12 582	18 872
	300/300	0.6	3 539	7 007	10 616
	400/400	0.8	1 992	3 984	5 976

CO_2 laser surgery in the oral cavity

30 W, the maximum power density is just over 10 000 W/cm². The handpiece beam is, therefore, about eight times more powerful than the microscope beam and although it has the disadvantage that dissection is not under magnified control, excision with the handpiece is more rapid. On the other hand, where accurate dissection rather than a powerful beam is required, such as for surface leukoplakia, the magnified image with the operating microscope allows more accurate control, with minimal damage to deeper tissues.

(c) Duration of exposure

The depth of penetration of the laser beam into the tissue depends not only on the spot size and the power density but also on the duration of exposure. This may be varied as a single or repeat pulsed beam or a continuous mode. In the oral cavity the repeat pulse mode is used initially to map out the line of the proposed excision and then the continuous beam can be used either for vaporization or excision (Figures 5.3 and 5.4).

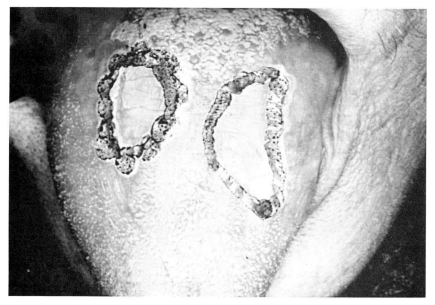

Figure 5.3 Two areas of leukoplakia on the dorsum of the tongue initially outlined with the laser.

Use of the CO_2 laser in the mouth

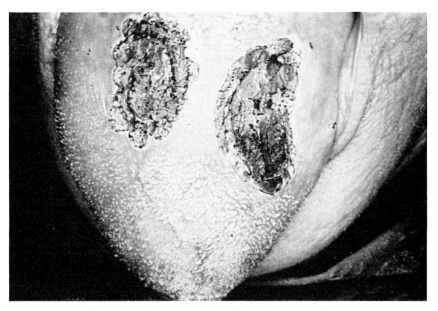

Figure 5.4 Appearance following laser excision.

5.3.2 TISSUE VARIABLES

The mucosal surface of the upper aerodigestive tract, particularly the oral cavity, is ideal for CO_2 laser therapy, but the complex contours and variations in texture of the mucosa make it sometimes a difficult area to treat predictably. Several factors relating to the type of lesion and tissue surface being treated should be considered prior to surgery because these may influence the choice of handpiece or microscope.

(a) Site and accessibility

The lips, the labial commissures and the anterior part of the tongue and alveolus are readily accessible to both the microscope and handpiece. Where excision, rather than vaporization is required the handpiece is easier and less cumbersome to use but in the posterior region of the mouth the microscope is preferable. The base of the tongue is particularly inaccessible even using a mouth gag and the laryngoscope is normally required. As previously mentioned, at this distance the power density is limited and excision of a large bulky lesion in the tongue base can be time consuming. Nevertheless, we have found the laser very suitable for hypertrophied lingual tonsils which can be resected with minimal bleeding.

107

CO_2 laser surgery in the oral cavity

(b) Tissue surface

Penetration of the CO_2 laser beam into the tissue surface will depend on the concentration of water in the cellular and extracellular components. The mucosal lining of the oral cavity varies in texture and thickness and in its susceptibility to laser vaporization. The thickly keratinized dorsal surface of the tongue has a relatively low water content and is, therefore, more resistant to the laser beam. Its carbon content is correspondingly higher and charring is more noticeable. The buccal or floor of mouth mucosa, however, is thin and is much more easily vaporized, whereas cortical bone and tooth enamel contain very little water and charring may result in permanent damage (Fisher and Frame, 1984).

Pathological lesions of the oral mucosa also vary considerably in texture. Oral leukoplakia in particular can be very misleading in its appearance and thickness. Highly keratinized lesions are best excised because surface vaporization may not completely eradicate the basal layers and regrowth is likely to occur.

(c) Size of lesion

Eradication of large surface lesions such as leukoplakia on the buccal mucosa, tongue and floor of mouth is preferably best carried out using microscopic control. Magnification of the operative field allows good visual control of dissection and suspicious areas are more readily identified. The depth of penetration can also be more easily monitored and unnecessary damage to underlying tissue is avoided.

(d) Depth of lesion

Benign surface lesions can be accurately excised with the laser using microscopic control if necessary. This is particularly helpful for haemangiomas where deep prolongations of the lesion, which might otherwise be missed and cause recurrence, can be readily identified and dissected in a bloodless field. Deeper resections are more easily carried out with the handpiece which can be used like the cutting diathermy and avoids cumbersome use of the microscope.

(e) Excision or vaporization?

As a basic surgical principle it is better to excise rather than destroy a lesion which is being removed, especially where the histological nature is uncertain. With a benign growth which is inaccessible to excision, vaporization is an acceptable alternative.

Healing of laser wounds of oral mucosa

In summary, the choice of the handpiece or operating microscope depends to a certain extent on availability and personal preference. However, consideration should be given to these variable factors so that the surgeon can optimize the advantages that the laser possesses in surgical treatment of oral cavity lesions.

5.4 Healing of laser wounds of oral mucosa

5.4.1 CLINICAL ASPECT

The CO_2 laser beam has a wavelength of 10.6 μm and is absorbed by water, resulting in vaporization of the intra- and extracellular fluid and rupture of the cell membranes (Hall *et al.*, 1971; Hall, Hill and Beach, 1971). The cellular particles are released into the laser beam where they are burnt up producing incandescence, and deposited as a carbonized layer on the wound surface. This surface layer appears to act as a protective covering and a dressing is not required. The oral mucosa generally has a high water content and many oral lesions are suitable for CO_2 laser excision. There are no viable cells within the released vapour and debris is not scattered into the adjacent tissue. In addition, there is no increased tendency to lymphatic or haematological spread of malignant cells (Mihashi *et al.*, 1976). The destructive effect of the CO_2 laser on soft tissue is localized, and there is an extremely narrow zone of damaged cells between the lasered area and the adjacent normal tissue. At the time of surgery there is minimal bleeding due to the laser sealing blood vessels less than 0.5 mm diameter; larger vessels are dealt with in the conventional manner. This allows the surgeon excellent visibility and precision when dissecting through the tissue planes.

Within 24 h, a fibrinous coagulum begins to form on the wound surface with a typical thick creamy yellow appearance and persists for several weeks. An interesting feature is the lack of swelling, inflammation or erythema of the surrounding tissues and a distinct boundary is evident between the treated area and adjacent epithelium. The oral mucosal wounds are slow to re-epithelialize and after one or two weeks new epithelium begins proliferating at the margins. Superficial mucosal wounds exhibit little contraction, and when re-epithelialization is complete after four to six weeks, the original outline of the wound is often still evident. The area feels soft on palpation and there is usually little postoperative scarring. Resection of a large bulk of soft tissue, such as in a partial glossectomy, is associated with slightly greater wound contraction and some scarring.

Laser surgery in the oral cavity is accomplished with little upset to the

CO_2 laser surgery in the oral cavity

patient, who has minimal pain immediately postoperatively. However, pain may be experienced three to four days after surgery and persist for one to two weeks. This discomfort is usually mild and is relieved by simple analgesics. Nevertheless, patients should be warned about the possibility of the late onset of pain, to avoid concern that some complication has occurred.

5.4.2 BIOLOGICAL ASPECTS

Comparative histological studies of wound healing following CO_2 laser and conventional surgical excision of buccal mucosa have been carried out in Birmingham (Fisher et al., 1983; Fisher and Frame, 1984). The changes following removal of 2 cm discs of oral mucosa using the two techniques were studied in an animal model over a period of 42 days. Visual inspection revealed satisfactory healing without infection, although the two types of wounds behaved differently. The surgically excised areas contracted considerably and had rolled margins which became flatter with time, but scarring was still visible at 48 days. The laser wounds initially had a buff-coloured base with adherent carbonized tissue fragments. Subsequently, there was little contraction and the edge of the wound was level with the adjacent tissue from an early stage.

The histological studies indicated that the surface of the laser wounds was composed of a layer of homogeneous basophilic coagulum beneath which was a narrow zone where the coagulum showed altered staining with eosin. In some superficial areas, desiccated brown coagulum was present. A fibrinous coagulum accumulated on the surface during the first few days, and was thickest after seven days. The acute inflammatory reaction reached its maximum after four days and was only mild. Epithelial cell migration was apparent at four days and continued until completed at 28 days. The process of epithelial cell migration over the damaged surface seemed to be less well controlled than in the surgical defects, and in most specimens areas of fibrinous coagulum were covered by the epithelium at the edges of the wound. In healing by secondary intention in conventional wounds, the epithelial cells normally proliferate along the boundary between the surface coagulum and the underlying granulation tissue. Few myofibroblasts were present beneath the lasered surface, in contrast to the large numbers in the surgical sites (Figures 5.5 and 5.6). After the completion of epithelialization at 28 days, a thin band of myofibroblasts was present beneath the epithelium across the full width of the wound. These cells were fewer at 42 days, when there was some reformation of collagen.

The differences between the laser and scalpel wounds in the oral

Healing of laser wounds of oral mucosa

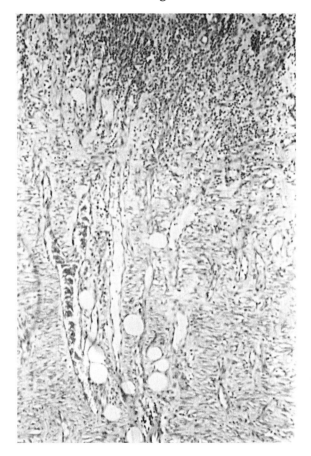

Figure 5.5 Scalpel wound at 7 days showing vertical capillary formation and horizontal sheets of myofibroblasts. At the top, just below the wound surface, there is an intense inflammatory cell infiltrate (H&E ×64).

mucosa were significant. The zone of tissue damage adjacent to the laser defects was narrow, and is probably related to the mechanism of tissue destruction. Vaporization of fluid and destruction of the cells might not release the chemical mediators of inflammation. The denatured collagen on the surface of the lasered area probably forms an impermeable layer in the immediate postoperative period and reduced the degree of tissue irritation from the oral contents. These factors probably account for the smaller inflammatory reaction in the laser wounds. The minimal degree of contraction following laser therapy is probably a consequence of the small numbers of myofibroblasts present. These cells are thought to be the effectors of wound contraction (Gabbiani, Ryan and Majno, 1971;

CO_2 laser surgery in the oral cavity

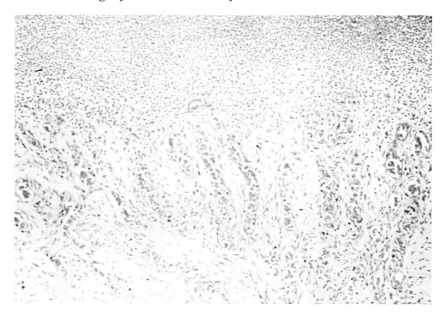

Figure 5.6 Laser wound at 14 days showing proliferation of capillaries and small number of randomly orientated myofibroblasts (H&E ×64).

Montandon, D'Andiran and Gabbiani, 1977). Following surgical excision with the scalpel, myofibroblasts were present in large numbers parallel to the surface so that contraction in their longitudinal axis resulted in reduction in the size of the defect. In contrast, only a few myofibroblasts were seen following laser treatment and these were largely restricted to the newly constituted lamina propria after each part of the wound had been re-epithelialized. In addition, their distribution lacked orientation, and thus their contraction would have little effect on the overall dimensions of the defect. The reason for the small number of myofibroblasts in these superficial laser wounds is not clear although it is probably related to the minor degree of tissue irritation. The lack of contraction may account for the delay in complete re-epithelialization when compared to scalpel defects because the surface area to be covered is greater.

The effects of the CO_2 laser on other oral tissues have also been investigated (Fisher and Frame, 1984). The removal of epithelium in the floor of the mouth around the orifices of the submandibular salivary gland duct produced no visible evidence of obstruction of salivary flow, with no swellings in the floor of mouth or submandibular regions. Histological studies showed that there was no stenosis of the ducts, and that the epithelium of the floor of mouth and duct orifices regenerated completely without any narrowing or distortion of the opening. Histological sections of the submandibular salivary glands confirmed that no obstructive changes had occurred in the glandular tissue. A similar healing pattern has been observed in patients who have undergone laser removal of lesions in the floor of mouth; none of the patients has reported symptoms of salivary obstruction or swelling of the submandibular salivary glands. This makes the CO_2 laser particularly useful for vaporizing patches of leukoplakia in the floor of mouth where the mucosa can be removed in the region of the submandibular salivary gland ducts without producing postoperative problems of duct stenosis. Sublingual keratosis is a lesion of considerable clinical importance because of the risk of malignant change (Kramer, El-Labban and Lee, 1978), and can be eliminated using the CO_2 laser.

Care must be taken when using the CO_2 laser to remove soft tissue overlying the mandible to avoid damaging the underlying cortical bone. This may result in chronic inflammation of the soft tissue and delayed healing. After radiotherapy the underlying bone may become necrotic with subsequent sequestration of devitalized fragments. Accidental contact of the CO_2 laser beam with the teeth causes craters involving the enamel and dentine, and there may be damage to the tooth pulps, even after a short laser impact.

The histological studies and clinical experience indicate that the CO_2 laser offers many advantages both to the patient and surgeon in the management of lesions of the oral soft tissues. Since 1981 more than 200 patients have been treated in Birmingham for laser removal of a wide range of oral pathology, either benign, premalignant or malignant. The distribution of the lesions is given in Table 5.3, and the type of pathology indicated in Table 5.4. It can be seen that leukoplakia accounted for three times as many lesions as benign or malignant types.

Table 5.3 Distribution of oral lesions treated with the laser

Tongue (anterior two-thirds)	84
Floor of mouth/lower alveolus	89
Cheek	38
Lips/commissures	26
Palate/upper alveolus	18
Total	255

CO_2 laser surgery in the oral cavity

Table 5.4 Pathology of lesions treated with the laser

Benign	58
'Leukoplakia'	146
Malignant	51
Total	255

5.5 Anaesthetic and safety aspects: special considerations in the oral cavity

The CO_2 laser is a potentially lethal instrument and nowhere is this fact more relevant than in the upper aerodigestive tract. The anaesthetist and surgeon must always work in close cooperation to safeguard the airway and to allow optimum surgical conditions. In the oral cavity most laser procedures are best carried out under general anaesthesia although small lesions around the lips and anterior tongue may be excised under local anaesthesia in suitable patients. When local anaesthesia is used it is difficult to prevent the patient moving inadvertently which may cause an accidental burn. They may become alarmed by the noise and vapour from the laser and may also object to having their face covered with the moistened protective dressing.

Where general anaesthesia is administered for anterior oral cavity lesions, a conventional nasal tube can be used provided that adequate protective moistened wool padding is placed securely around the tube before it enters the nose, and that the posterior part of the oral cavity is packed with moistened gauze to safeguard the tube in the oropharynx.

Alternative protected methods of intubation are required for lesions elsewhere in the oral cavity and these include:

1. endotracheal tube covered with aluminium tape;
2. flexible metal endotracheal tube;
3. laser resistant endotracheal tube.

These methods and other safety measures are discussed in detail in Chapter 1.

5.6 Treatment of oral lesions

The surgeon has a choice of two techniques when removing lesions in the mouth with the CO_2 laser, either excision or vaporization. As a general rule it is preferable to excise the lesion because this provides

Treatment of oral lesions

histological evidence of its complete removal and confirmation of the diagnosis. During vaporization there is a risk that small fragments of the lesion may not be eliminated by the laser beam. In addition, soft tissues with a highly keratinized surface are resistant to vaporization because of their low water content, and these are better excised. If a pathological lesion is vaporized, it is important that a biopsy is obtained either pre-operatively or at the time of lasering.

5.6.1 BENIGN LESIONS

A review is presented of the first 40 patients who underwent removal of 43 benign oral lesions using the CO_2 laser, either the Coherent 450 or the Sharplan 733 machines (Frame, 1985).

There were 22 males and 18 females, with an age range of 12–67 years (mean, 48.6 years). The histology of the conditions is shown in Table 5.5. The therapy was performed under general anaesthesia because this was less upsetting to the patients and they were less likely to move unintentionally during the procedure. In addition, the lesions were often widespread in the mouth. Small lesions suitable for excision under local anaesthetic were not included in this series because they were treated by conventional techniques.

(a) Denture-induced hyperplasia

This usually presents as areas of fibro-epithelial hyperplasia in the upper or lower labial sulcus, associated with the periphery of an unstable denture which has caused long-term trauma to the mucosa. If the mass of soft tissue is excised with the scalpel, there may be difficulty in obtaining primary closure of the resultant defect, and healing may be complicated by contraction and scarring. This can result in loss of sulcus

Table 5.5 Histology of 43 benign lesions removed with CO_2 laser

Denture induced hyperplasia	16
Mucous cyst/ranula	9
Pleomorphic adenoma	5
Papilloma	4
Pyogenic granuloma	3
Fibro-epithelial polyp	3
Haemangioma	2
Fibroma	1
Total	43

CO_2 laser surgery in the oral cavity

depth and lead to subsequent problems with denture retention. A split-thickness skin graft may be applied to the raw area to minimize this complication. Cryotherapy has been recommended for these lesions (Leopard and Poswillo, 1974), but the procedure is time consuming and is followed by considerable swelling. The CO_2 laser has been found to be a precise method of excising large denture granulomas with little upset to the patient afterwards. Following re-epithelialization of the wound, the lasered area feels soft on palpation with little distortion of the soft tissues, and patients do not have problems in wearing dentures afterwards.

(b) Mucous cyst and ranula

A mucous cyst is a thin-walled, bluish, fluctuant swelling occurring just beneath the oral mucosa and filled with mucoid material. It usually appears after damage to a minor salivary gland following which there is extravasation of mucus into the tissues, or occasionally it forms from dilatation of the duct of a minor salivary gland. In the floor of the mouth it often arises from the sublingual salivary gland and is known as a ranula. The lining consists of a thin layer of condensed fibrous tissue, and only rarely is epithelium present. The accepted treatment of a mucous cyst is excision of the sac and the associated minor salivary gland with the scalpel, or elimination using the cryoprobe. However, it occasionally recurs or becomes persistent, and in this situation the CO_2 laser is an ideal means of vaporizing the soft tissue lesion. Following this therapy, there is little contraction or scarring, and this is obviously of importance in areas such as the lower lip which is a common site for these cysts to occur. A ranula is treated by exposure and removal of the sublingual salivary gland, together with the associated soft tissue sac (Catone, Merrill and Henny, 1969). However, during excision the ranula is frequently ruptured and subsequent dissection of the cyst sac may be difficult. An advantage of the CO_2 laser is that it will vaporize the cyst sac and destroy all of the residual pathological tissue. The procedure is relatively bloodless and allows the surgeon good visibility in the potentially vascular area of the floor of the mouth. The laser may also be utilized for dissection and excision of the sublingual salivary gland, after which the wound is left to re-epithelialize. The patients have reported little discomfort following surgery and have regained full oral function.

(c) Pleomorphic adenoma

This is the commonest tumour of the palate and arises from a minor salivary gland. It often occurs at the junction of the hard and soft

Treatment of oral lesions

palates, frequently to one side of the mid-line. The tumour is excised with a margin of healthy tissue to avoid the risk of recurrence. Local enucleation usually results in tumour cells being left behind because of the nature of the lesion:

1. the capsule at the periphery is often incomplete;
2. there is a tendency for a split to occur within the tumour tissue beneath the capsule;
3. there are frequently localized outgrowths of tumour cells through the capsule.

Adequate surgical excision may necessitate full thickness resection of the soft palate with communication into the nasopharynx. The resultant palatal fenestration is managed by surgical repair or by prosthetic means. Excision of a pleomorphic adenoma of the soft palate using the CO_2 laser has several advantages. At the time of surgery, the operator has excellent visibility and control of haemorrhage, which facilitate accurate resection of the lesion with a suitable margin of healthy tissue. The surgeon can visualize the tissue planes through which he is dissecting and avoids the risk of cutting too close to the tumour. Following re-epithelialization of the wound, the tissues remain soft and pliable, without restriction or mobility of the soft palate. Because of the

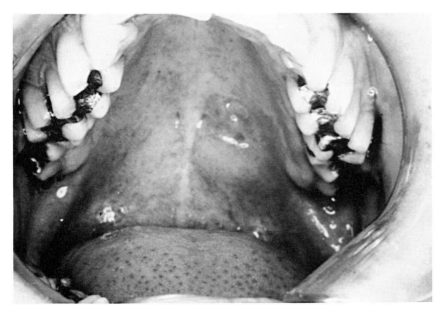

Figure 5.7 Pleomorphic adenoma at junction of hard and soft palate on left side.

CO_2 laser surgery in the oral cavity

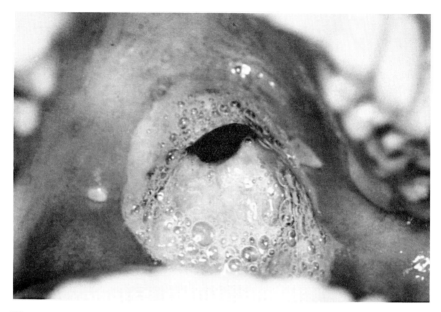

Figure 5.8 Five days after laser excision showing fibrinous coagulum and oronasal communication.

excellent healing and regeneration after CO_2 laser surgery, small palatal fenestrations of about 1 cm in diameter often heal spontaneously, and larger areas reduce in size (Figures 5.7–5.9). There is minimal scarring, and any residual oronasal communication can be readily closed using a rotation flap.

(d) Miscellaneous benign lesions

A variety of other benign swellings in the mouth have been removed using the CO_2 laser. This form of treatment is especially beneficial when the lesion is large, potentially vascular, or situated in the posterior region of the mouth. Following surgery, the areas healed well without complications.

Although many small benign lesions in the mouth can be easily excised with a scalpel under local anaesthesia, the CO_2 laser does have a place in the treatment of certain benign lesions and offers an alternative therapy for selected patients.

5.6.2 PREMALIGNANT LESIONS

The number of different types of these lesions removed with the CO_2 laser is shown in Table 5.6.

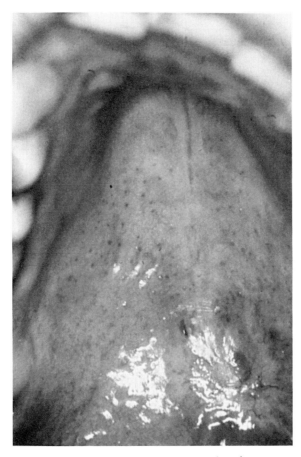

Figure 5.9 Spontaneous healing 4 months after treatment.

Table 5.6 Oral premalignant lesions removed with the CO_2 laser

Chronic hyperplastic candidiasis (candidal leukoplakia)	6
Erosive lichen planus	7
Leukoplakia Hyperkeratosis mild dysplasia moderate dysplasia severe dysplasia	129
Carcinoma in situ	4
Total	146

CO_2 laser surgery in the oral cavity

(a) Leukoplakia

The CO_2 laser possesses many advantages as a means of eliminating intra-epithelial pathology in the mouth. The most important oral pre-malignant lesion is leukoplakia which is defined as 'a white patch that cannot be assigned on the basis of clinical or laboratory findings to any other diagnostic category' (Pindborg et al., 1963). This lesion is considered to be potentially premalignant because progression to invasive squamous cell carcinoma at the same site may occur in a small number of cases. Initial biopsy and histological examination are essential to assess its true nature. Epithelial dyskeratosis or cellular atypia denote disordered proliferation, maturation and organization of the epithelium and are taken as the prognostic guides of premalignancy. White patches exhibiting these features behave, however, in an unpredictable manner and, although some may progress to invasive squamous cell carcinoma, others remain static for years while a few may even regress. The incidence of malignant change has been reviewed by Cawson (1975), Kramer (1976) and Pindborg (1980) who quoted studies in which the transformation rates ranged from 0.13% to 6%. Although these figures are low, patients with this condition have a likelihood of developing oral cancer which is 50–100 times greater than the rest of the population (Einhorn and Wersall, 1967).

Two clinical features of oral leukoplakia are important in relation to the chance of malignant transformation, namely colour change and the site in the mouth. 'Leukoplakia' with a red, velvety appearance (erythroplakia) is a high-risk lesion (Banoczy and Sugar, 1972). Speckled leukoplakia, which is a combination of white and red areas and may be associated with a chronic candidal infection (Pindborg, 1971), also has a high incidence of malignant change. The position of the patch of leukoplakia in the mouth is also important, with the floor of mouth and ventral surface on the tongue being most at risk (Kramer, El-Labban and Lee, 1978).

(b) Other oral premalignant lesions

Chronic hyperplastic candidiasis (or candidal leukoplakia) is a thickened raised white patch associated with chronic candidal infection, but differs from other types of candidiasis is that it is adherent and cannot be wiped off. Epithelial hyperplasia may be gross and there may be cellular atypia (Cawson, 1966). These lesions sometimes undergo malignant change (Cawson and Lehner, 1968; Eyre and Nally, 1971). A common cause of white patches on the oral mucosa is lichen planus which usually presents as a lace-like network of raised white striae on

Treatment of oral lesions

the inner aspect of the cheeks or the dorsum of the tongue. It is often symptomless, although the atrophic and erosive forms may be painful. Carcinoma develops in lichen planus only rarely, and is more likely to do so in the atrophic types (Kovesi and Banoczy, 1973).

(c) Management

Patches of candidal leukoplakia are treated with topical antifungal drugs but are often persistent. Lichen planus requires therapy only when symptoms are produced due to erosion or ulceration, and often responds to topical cortisteroids. The management of oral leukoplakia depends on the histology, clinical appearance, and site in the mouth. If the surgeon considers that a patch of leukoplakia should be eliminated, then the CO_2 laser has many advantages compared to other forms of treatment. Since 1981, 146 premalignant patches have been eliminated in the mouth using CO_2 laser (Frame *et al.*, 1984; Rhys Evans, Frame and Brandrick, 1986). A biopsy was obtained either pre-operatively or, in a few cases, at the time of laser treatment. Two techniques were employed: excision of the affected epithelium together with some of the underlying soft tissue or vaporization of the area. In both situations the tissue to be eliminated was initially outlined with the laser beam to mark clearly the boundaries. Excision is a better technique because it allows the surgeon to remove the entire affected area of epithelium and some of the underlying connective tissue. The elimination of this deeper layer may reduce the likelihood of recurrence of leukoplakia because investigations of malignant lesions have indicated that the subepithelial tissues may play a role in the induction of such disease (Smith, 1980). Another advantage of excision is that the patch of epithelium is available for serial histological examination to verify the nature of the lesion and identify any areas of increased cellular activity, or early invasion. A potential problem with vaporization of a patch of abnormal mucosa is that small fragments may not be eliminated by the laser, resulting in rapid recurrence. In addition, mucosal lesions with a thick, highly keratinized surface are resistant to vaporization because of the low water content. However, there are certain areas of the mouth where access is restricted and it may be difficult to excise a patch of abnormal epithelium with the CO_2 laser; in this situation the patch may be vaporized.

The seven patients with erosive lichen planus were treated because they had experienced persistent discomfort despite long-term therapy with topical medicaments, and the six patients with candidal leukoplakia had not responded to anti-fungal drugs. The 129 patches of oral leukoplakia varied histologically from hyperkeratosis to severe epithelial dysplasia. Four patches of carcinoma in situ have been excised with the CO_2 laser.

(d) Follow up

Healing following laser removal of the oral mucosal lesions generally progressed well. There was little wound contraction, even at sites such as the commissure of the mouth or the ventral surface of the tongue. Re-epithelialization was complete after four to six weeks and the new epithelium appeared healthy in most patients. There was little post-operative scarring or distortion of the soft tissues which felt soft on palpation (Figures 5.10 and 5.11). In a few elderly patients, the regenerated epithelium appeared rather thin and atrophic and in one patient the outline of the wound could still be seen even after two years.

The CO_2 laser is probably not suitable for treating erosive lichen planus or candidal leukoplakia because of the rapid recurrence of the lesions. Five of the patches of the erosive lichen planus and three areas of candidal leukoplakia recurred within a period of two years after treatment. However, several of the patients reported that their mouths were less painful than before laser therapy. The patients who were treated with the CO_2 laser for elimination of patches of oral leukoplakia

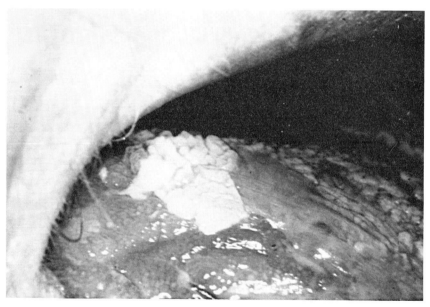

Figure 5.10 Area of leukoplakia on right lateral border of the tongue.

Treatment of oral lesions

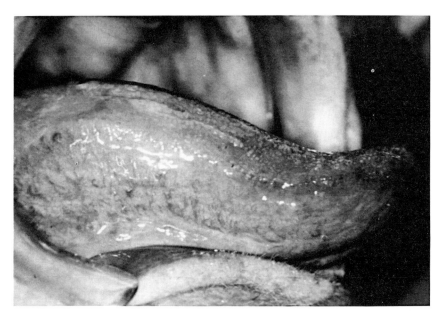

Figure 5.11 Appearance 4 months after laser treatment showing re-epithelialization of the wound.

progressed much more satisfactorily. At present, a long-term follow-up is under way to assess the recurrence rate and to obtain a comparison with scalpel excision and cryotherapy. Initial results indicate that the recurrence rate is low (Frame *et al.*, 1984; Rhys Evans, Frame and Brandrick, 1986). However, it should be remembered that the CO_2 laser does not have any greater ability than the scalpel to 'cure' these conditions; rather it is a precise means of eliminating soft tissue pathology with little upset to the patient afterwards. Following the treatment, the acute inflammatory reaction is minimal, and there is little swelling or oedema. Healing generally is excellent and, because of the limited contraction and scarring that occurs, there is little restriction in mobility of the soft tissues or interference with oral function. Patients who have leukoplakia in the mouth often have generalized instability of the oral epithelium and healthy looking mucosa adjacent to a white patch may have undergone dysplastic changes. Following the excision of leukoplakia by any type of surgery, the new epithelium that migrates from the periphery to cover the wound may originate from an area of potentially unstable mucosa and rapidly undergo dysplastic changes. An advantage of the CO_2 laser in the management of leukoplakia is that the reduced contraction and scarring means that a recurrence can be treated without producing severe restriction in mobility of the soft tissue.

5.6.3 MALIGNANT LESIONS

(a) Indications for laser surgery

The introduction of the carbon dioxide laser in recent years has rekindled interest in transoral resection of tumours of the upper aerodigestive tract. In the past this was a well-established method of managing oral cavity cancer (Whitehead, 1981) but its popularity waned during the mid part of this century when a more aggressive approach to these lesions was generally adopted. External composite resections were advocated, often sacrificing the mandible, but at the same time great advances in reconstructive techniques allowed better restoration of function.

Recent advances in anaesthesia, airway control, frozen section techniques and the use of the CO_2 laser have provided more suitable conditions for precise surgical excision of oral cavity tumours. The laser does not possess any greater potential of curing cancer compared with conventional surgical techniques and the survival rate of patients will depend largely on the ability of the surgeon to deliver a specimen with histologically clear margins (Strong *et al.*, 1979). Excision of infiltrating tumours must follow accepted oncological principles with adequate margins of clearance under visual control, palpation and frozen section confirmation. Usually at least a 1 cm margin is required, but for tongue tumours especially following radiotherapy, evidence suggests that this is inadequate and should be extended to at least 2 cm (Harrison, 1983). The high incidence of local recurrence despite histologically negative margins is in the region of 32–36% (Harrison, 1983; Looser, Shah and Strong, 1978) and confirms the necessity for wide clearance of tongue tumours not only on the surface but also in the deeper muscular plane.

With these limitations in mind, the surgeon should be able to define the indications for transoral laser excision. Small and medium-sized tumours are suitable if they are accessible and, if situated in the tongue, should be limited to the mobile anterior two thirds. Extension into the base of the tongue will necessitate a lateral pharyngotomy approach or composite transmandibular resection. The laser can also be used effectively in palliation of painful ulcerating tumours which can be resected with minimal morbidity.

(b) Surgical technique

For transoral resections the lesion and surrounding tissue should be stabilized with stay sutures and dissection carried out in an antero-

Treatment of oral lesions

posterior direction either with the handpiece or microscope (Figures 5.12 and 5.13). Great care must be taken to protect the lips and face with moist gauze to prevent accidental burns. The handpiece has the advantage of more rapid dissection because the smaller spot size has a power density which is more than seven times greater than with the microscope using a 300 mm lens. The handpiece is also less cumbersome than the microscope which has to be moved frequently to keep it in focus. Nevertheless, Carruth (1982) has shown in a large series of tongue resections that the use of the laser microscope is entirely satisfactory.

With the larger oral cavity tumour where composite resection including radical neck dissection and hemimandibulectomy is necessary, the place of the laser is questionable. It will facilitate dissection of the

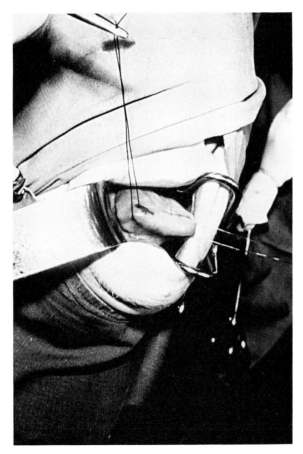

Figure 5.12 Squamous carcinoma of right side of tongue. Stay suture to anchor tissue prior to hemiglossectomy.

CO_2 laser surgery in the oral cavity

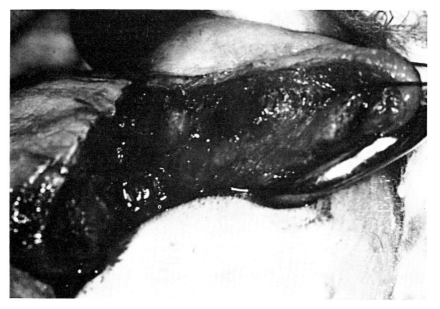

Figure 5.13 Hemiglossectomy proceeding with minimal bleeding.

tongue, but when this is just a small part of a larger radical resection, the advantage gained by use of the laser is less significant and may not be time-saving. It is also unsuitable for resection of bone which is more easily carried out using a saw or osteotome, and is certainly inadvisable in the deeper tissues of the neck. A temporary tracheostomy is preferable for composite resections and occasionally for deep excisions involving the mid-third portion of the tongue.

(c) Reconstruction following laser excision

Experimental evidence has shown that following excision of superficial oral cavity lesions, re-epithelialization is accomplished with minimal contracture (Fisher *et al.*, 1983; Fisher and Frame, 1984). Complete healing of the wound contraction leaves a wide area to epithelialize. Clinical experience has confirmed these findings and lesions can be excised without the need for skin grafts or pedicle flaps (Carruth, 1983; Rhys Evans, Frame and Brandrick, 1986). Animal model experiments have also shown that with deeper excisions of the tongue some recovery of tongue volume is achieved.

Anterior partial glossectomies and resection of buccal and floor of mouth lesions can be carried out with minimal disturbance of function

Treatment of oral lesions

(Figure 5.14) and there is little need for prolonged stay in hospital. Large excisions of the cheek mucosa including buccinator and the buccal pad of fat require reconstruction, for which we have found the radial free skin graft satisfactory. Wide resections involving the tongue base require replacement of the tissue and lining defect with a myocutaneous or similar flap (Rhys Evans and Das Gupta, 1980). Early restoration of the velopharyngeal sphincter at the tongue base is essential for re-establishment of the swallowing mechanism.

Table 5.7 gives a summary of 51 tumours excised with the laser, the majority (44) of which were squamous cell carcinomas. Long-term

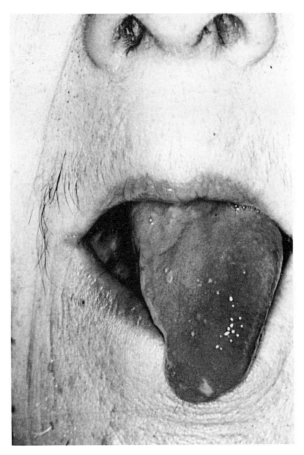

Figure 5.14 Appearance of tongue 1 week after surgery showing good mobility and minimal oedema.

CO_2 laser surgery in the oral cavity

Table 5.7 Malignant lesions

Lymphoma	1
Adenoid cystic carcinoma	2
Squamous cell carcinoma	44
Adenocarcinoma	3
Osteogenic sarcoma	1
Total	51

follow-up is being evaluated but nine recurrences (20%) have been recorded which is similar to other published series.

5.7 Complications of CO_2 laser surgery

In comparison with other methods of treating oral cavity lesions, the laser is safe and complications are relatively few provided that care is taken with surgical technique and that the laser safety code is strictly followed (Carruth, McKenzie and Wainwright, 1980). Problems which may arise can be classified as immediate, early or late.

5.7.1 IMMEDIATE

1. Accidental burn to patient's lips, soft tissues or teeth.
2. Accidental burn to surgeon or theatre staff.
3. Anaesthetic tube combustion and airway complications.

5.7.2 EARLY POSTOPERATIVE

(a) Pain

This is usually minimal or absent but some patients complain of discomfort after the second or third day. At the time of surgery, the laser causes minimal damage to adjacent tissue and immediately afterwards, a surface coagulum covers and seals the wound. These factors delay and minimize the inflammatory reaction and release of vaso- and neuroactive substances normally associated with stimulation of nerve endings. Carruth (1982) stressed the low morbidity and lack of postoperative pain in his series of tongue resections. With treatment of surface leukoplakias we have found that postoperative discomfort is more variable.

Complications of CO_2 laser surgery

(b) Haemorrhage

Bleeding at the time of operation is minimal but care must be taken especially in tongue resections to ligate branches of the lingual artery which may be the cause of reactionary haemorrhage.

(c) Granuloma

In three patients treated for lesions on the lateral aspect of the tongue small granulomatous swellings developed in the centre of the healing area and delayed healing (Figure 5.15). Excision revealed that the ingrowing epithelium had become trapped beneath a central raised area of granulation tissue (Figure 5.16). The lateral border of the tongue may be particularly prone to this problem because of repeated trauma from the teeth. Simple removal of the granuloma was followed by complete healing of the wound.

5.7.3 LATE POSTOPERATIVE

(a) Scarring

Minimal scarring occurs following superficial excisions but certain conditions will predispose to increased formation of scar tissue, espe-

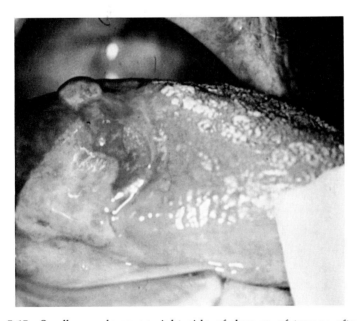

Figure 5.15 Small granuloma on right side of dorsum of tongue after laser treatment.

CO_2 laser surgery in the oral cavity

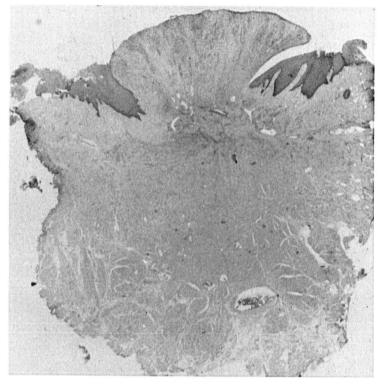

Figure 5.16 Histology of excised lesion shows a granuloma with the migrating epithelial edges growing underneath it preventing complete healing.

cially with deeper resection. These include previous radiotherapy or surgery and submucous fibrosis.

(b) Veloglossal incompetence

This may occur following wide resections of the middle and posterior third of the tongue if lost tissue is not replaced. In such cases normal swallowing may be delayed for up to three months.

(c) Recurrence

Although the laser facilitates accurate excision of soft tissue pathology in the mouth there are other factors which predispose to the recurrence of premalignant and malignant lesions.

References

Banoczy, J. and Sugar, L. (1972), Longitudinal studies in oral leukoplakia. *J. Oral Pathol.*, **1**, 265–72.

Carruth, J. A. S. (1982), Resection of the tongue with the carbon dioxide laser. *J. Laryngol. Otol.*, **96**, 529–43.

Carruth, J. A. S. (1983), Lasers in head and neck cancer. In *Head and Neck Cancer* (eds P. H. Rhys Evans, P. E. Robin and J. W. L. Fielding), Castle House Publications, Tunbridge Wells, pp. 136–50.

Carruth, J. A. S., McKenzie, A. L. and Wainwright, A. C. (1980), The carbon dioxide laser: safety aspects. *J. Laryngol. Otol.*, **94**, 411–17.

Catone, G. A., Merrill, R. G. and Henny, F. A. (1969), Sublingual gland mucus-escape phenomenon: treatment by excision of the sublingual gland. *J. Oral Surg.*, **27**, 774–86.

Cawson, R. A. (1966), Chronic oral candidiasis and leukoplakia. *Oral Surg.*, **22**, 582–91.

Cawson, R. A. (1975), Premalignant lesions in the mouth. *Br. Med. Bull.*, **31**, 164–8.

Cawson, R. A. and Lehner, T. (1968), Chronic hyperplastic candidiasis – candidal leukoplakia. *Br. J. Dermatol.*, **80**, 9–16.

Einhorn, J. and Wersäll, J. (1967), Incidence of oral carcinoma in patients with leukoplakia of the oral mucosa. *Cancer*, **20**, 2189–93.

Eyre, J. and Nally, F. F. (1971), Oral candidosis and carcinoma. *Br. J. Dermatol.*, **85**, 73–5.

Fisher, S. E., Frame, J. W., Browne, R. M. and Tranter, R. M. D. (1983), A comparative histological study of wound healing following CO_2 laser and conventional surgical excision of canine buccal mucosa. *Arch. Oral Biol.*, **28**, 287–91.

Fisher, S. E. and Frame, J. W. (1984), The effects of the carbon dioxide surgical laser on oral tissues. *Br. J. Oral Maxillofac. Surg.*, **22**, 414–25.

Frame, J. W. (1985), Carbon dioxide laser surgery for benign oral lesions. *Br. Dent. J.*, **158**, 125–8.

Frame, J. W., Das Gupta, A. R., Dalton, G. A. and Rhys Evans, P. H. (1984), Use of the carbon dioxide laser in the management of premalignant lesions of the oral mucosa. *J. Laryngol. Otol.*, **98**, 1251–60.

Gabbiani, G., Ryan, G. B. and Majno, G. (1971), The presence of modified fibroblasts in granulation tissue and their possible role in wound contraction. *Experienta*, **27**, 549–50.

Hall, R. R., Beach, A. D., Baker, E. and Morison, P. C. A. (1971), Incision of tissue by carbon dioxide laser. *Nature Lond.*, **232**, 131–2.

Hall, R. R., Hill, D. W. and Beach, A. D. (1971), A carbon dioxide surgical laser. *Ann. R. Coll. Surg.*, **48**, 181–8.

Harrison, D. F. N. (1983), The questionable value of total glossectomy. *Head Neck Surg.*, **6**, 632–8.

Kovesi, G. and Banoczy, J. (1973), Follow-up studies in oral lichen planus. *Int. J. Oral Surg.*, **2**, 13–19.

Kramer, I. R. H. (1976) Precancerous lesions in the mouth. *J. Laryngol. Otol.*, **90**, 95–100.

Kramer, I. R. H., El-Labban, N. and Lee, K. W. (1978), The clinical features and risk of malignant transformation in sublingual keratosis. *Br. Dent. J.*, **144**, 171–80.

Leopard, P. J. and Poswillo, D. E. (1974), Practical cryosurgery for oral lesions. *Br. Dent. J.*, **136**, 185–96.

Looser, K. G., Shah, J. P. and Strong, E. W. (1978), The significance of positive margins in surgically resected epidermoid carcinomas. *Head Neck Surg.*, **1**, 107–11.

Mihashi, S., Jako, G. J., Incze, J., Strong, M. S. and Vaughan, C. W. (1976), Laser surgery in otolaryngology – interaction of CO_2 laser and soft tissue. *Ann. NY Acad. Sci.*, **267**, 263–94.

Montandon, D., D'Andiran, G. and Gabbiani, G. (1977), The mechanism of wound contraction and epithelialisation: clinical and experimental studies. *Clin. Plast. Surg.*, **4**, 325–46.

Pindborg, J. J. (1971), Oral leukoplakia. *Aust. Dent. J.*, **16**, 83–94.

Pindborg, J. J. (1980), *Oral Cancer and Precancer*. Bristol, Wright.

Pindborg, J. J., Renstrup, G., Poulsen, H. E. and Silverman, S. (1963), Studies in oral leukoplakia. *Acta Odont. Scand.*, **21**, 407–14.

Rhys Evans, P. H. and Das Gupta, A. R. (1981), The use of the pectoralis major myocutaneous flap for one-stage reconstruction of the base of the tongue. *J. Laryngol. Otol.*, **95**, 809.

Rhys Evans, P. H., Frame, J. W. and Brandrick, J. (1986), A review of carbon dioxide laser surgery in the oral cavity and pharynx. *J. Laryngol. Otol.*, **100**, 69–77.

Smith, C. J. (1980), Connective tissue influence on epithelial malignancy or premalignancy. In *Oral Premalignancy* (eds I. C. Mackenzie, E. Dabelsteen and C. A. Squier), University of Iowa Press, Iowa City.

Strong, M., Vaughan, C. W., Healy, G. B., Shapshay, S. M. and Jako, G. J. (1979), Transoral management of localised carcinoma of the oral cavity using the CO_2 laser. *Laryngoscope*, **89**, 897–905.

Whitehead, W. (1981), A hundred cases of entire excision of the tongue. *Br. Med. J.*, **1**, 961–5.

6 Micro-endoscopic CO_2 laser surgery of the hypopharyngeal diverticulum

J. J. M. VAN OVERBEEK

6.1 Aetiology, symptoms and diagnosis

Over the course of the years, many theories on the pathogenesis of hypopharyngeal diverticula have been put forward, but none of these has been generally accepted. There is agreement, however, on the site at which the diverticulum forms. This site is constant and found immediately above the oesophageal inlet on the posterior wall of the distal part of the hypopharynx. Between the propulsive oblique fibres of the inferior constrictor muscle and the horizontal fibres of the cricopharyngeus muscle with its sphincter function at the oesophageal inlet, there is a triangular area with only scanty muscle fibres. This weak spot – the triangle of Killian (1908) – is important in the pathogenesis. Anatomical studies in normal controls show the presence of local variations in the anatomy of the pharyngo-oesophageal segment; in some individuals there is a large triangle of Killian with a small mucosal herniation. As a result of pressure gradients the mucosa of the hypopharynx pouches out and at a later stage the mucosal prolapse forms the diverticular sac. At this level the food bolus has to be passed from the wide funnel-shaped hypopharynx through the relatively narrow oesophageal inlet.

By simultaneous intraluminal pressure recordings we have obtained sufficient information to reject the theory of a disorder in temporal coordination between hypopharynx and sphincter as a cause of diverticulum formation. We have also been unable to confirm the hypothesis of increased resting sphincter pressure or insufficient sphincter relaxation (Overbeek 1977).

It appears that an anatomical predisposition plays a prominent role in the mucosal herniation. This is also suggested by the familial incidence of these relatively rare diverticula. In our group of 413 patients we found a significant familial incidence. This series includes one family with three brothers, two families with two brothers and one male

Micro-endoscopic CO_2 laser surgery

patient in whose mother a Zenker's diverticulum was demonstrated radiologically. Age is undoubtedly of importance in the aetiology as pouches are rarely seen under the age of 40 years. There is no apparent reason for the fact that Zenker's diverticulum is more than twice as common in males as in females. However, the size of the laryngeal skeleton may explain this difference. The sex distribution in our group of patients is: 257 males and 156 females, with the age of the patients ranging from 33 to 94 years.

In many patients with a hypopharyngeal diverticulum the symptomatology is so characteristic as to be virtually pathognomonic: dysphagia, foetor oris, gurgling noises in the neck on swallowing, coughing and repeated infections of the bronchi due to aspiration. The duration of symptoms may range from a few weeks to many years.

The diagnosis of hypopharyngeal diverticulum is established by barium swallow and it is visible on lateral or in an oblique projection, but barium X-rays can show widely varying appearances in the same patient depending on the moment of exposure during swallowing.

It is generally assumed that chronic irritation and inflammation of the diverticular wall as a result of food retention are factors predisposing to carcinoma in a diverticulum. Data on the incidence vary, but it appears to be a rare complication with an incidence of 0.5% or even lower. In this series there have been two patients with carcinoma in the pouch in a total of 413 patients. One of these patients was treated by diverticulectomy and radiotherapy, and the other patient with radiotherapy and micro-endoscopic treatment of the pouch three months later.

6.2 Therapy

6.2.1 SURGICAL EXCISION

It is understandable that the first attempts to remove a hypopharyngeal diverticulum – at the end of the last century – carried a high mortality. It is probably for this reason that other methods of treatment were tried, e.g. invagination and diverticulopexy (surgical fixation of the floor of the diverticulum proximal to the diverticular entry).

After 1910, some surgeons began to suture the dissected diverticular sac to the skin or to the sternomastoid muscle with extirpation of the diverticulum at a second operation a few days later. This two-stage procedure, perfected by Lahey (1954), greatly reduced the much feared risk of mediastinitis. The introduction of antibiotics was one of the factors which contributed to an ever-increasing acceptance of one-stage diverticulectomy. The theory that the upper oesophageal sphincter (cricopharyngeus muscle) could be a factor in the aetiology of the

Therapy

diverticulum, persuaded surgeons to combine a diverticulectomy with an extra mucosal myotomy of this sphincter in an attempt to reduce the risk of recurrence.

As early as 1932, Seiffert (1932), performed myotomy of the sphincter in a patient with a walnut-sized diverticulum, which was itself left intact. He achieved complete disappearance of symptoms and repeated radiological follow-ups showed that the diverticulum was no longer demonstrable. Serles (1967), and Ellis et al. (1969), also reported good results. Although the exact aetiology of the hypopharyngeal diverticulum still remains to be established, it seems plausible that the combination of the triangle of Killian (as a weak spot in the hypopharyngeal wall) and the upper oesophageal sphincter localized immediately distal to it, are of importance in the pathogenesis of this pulsion diverticulum. Consequently it seems sensible not only to close the site of herniation after diverticulectomy, but also to eliminate the sphincter function by means of a myotomy.

6.2.2 ENDOSCOPIC TREATMENT

It is recognized that Mosher (1917) was the first to divide the septum between diverticulum and oesophagus under endoscopic control. Mosher wrote that he had for years entertained the idea of treating a hypopharyngeal diverticulum in this way. Initially he had refrained from using this method for fear of cutting vessels and nerves while dividing the tissue bridge, and for fear of possible mediastinitis after the operation. Anatomical studies however, taught him that no important structures were present in the septum. Mosher reported that owing to the position of the diverticulum in line with the hypopharynx, it could be difficult to find the displaced oesophageal inlet, and this is why he resorted to ballooning of the hypopharynx and the diverticulum. Once the oesophageal inlet was located it was dilated with the aid of probes and the oesophagoscope was so adjusted that the septum 'bisects the transverse diameter of the oesophagoscope', and scissors were then used to divide the spur strictly in the midline. In his publication Mosher mentioned four patients. In the first patient only a small cut was made in the spur; in the second it was cut halfway; in the third it was cut two-thirds of the way; and in the fourth, the entire tissue bridge was divided. None of the patients showed evidence of mediastinitis, and all showed complete improvement in symptoms. In view of these results, Mosher continued to use this method until, unfortunately, his seventh patient developed mediastinitis with a fatal outcome. He described this in the textbook of Jackson and Coates (1929), and in a separate publication (1935).

Micro-endoscopic CO_2 laser surgery

It was not until 1947 that another report on endoscopic treatment was published. Impressed with the results obtained by Seiffert (1932), in patients with a hypopharyngeal diverticulum treated exclusively by transcutaneous myotomy of the cricopharyngeus muscle. Schubel (1947), thought that a myotomy might just as well be performed endoscopically. He considered that the risk of mediastinitis was small in view of the presence of adhesions between the diverticulum and the posterior oesophageal wall. Moreover, he believed that after division of the septum the wound edges would separate, thus ensuring ample drainage of the pouch into the oesophagus, and he obtained good results in nine patients. To facilitate the location of the oesophageal inlet, Schubel had his patients swallow a long silk thread with a small lead pellet at the end a few days before the operation. Radiography usually showed that after one day the pellet had already reached the stomach or a more distal level of the digestive tract, and when the endoscope was introduced over the thread, the oesophageal inlet could quickly be found.

Dohlman (1949), described 39 patients with a hypopharyngeal diverticulum who he had treated endoscopically since 1935. He maintained that endoscopic treatment could be regarded as the treatment of choice if the cause of the diverticulum was in the cricopharyngeus muscle, as this procedure divided the sphincter and at the same time improved drainage from the diverticulum into the oesophagus. Dohlman also had his patients swallow a thread with a pellet before the operation, as he had often found it difficult to locate the oesophageal inlet. He developed a special set of instruments for this form of treatment and used an oesophagoscope with a divided end, inserting the upper lip into the oesophagus with the slightly shorter lower lip in the diverticulum with the spur as a horizontal tissue bar between the two parts of the oesophagoscope. He then injected local anaesthetic into the spur, and coagulated it in the midline with insulated diathermy forceps and then divided the coagulated tissue with a diathermy knife. Dohlman (1960), published a detailed account of his instruments and their application and described nearly 100 patients treated with them. Initially, he divided the spur in several stages in order to avoid unnecessary risks but gradually he carried out a complete division in one or two stages. Dohlman reported no serious postoperative complications and he believed that the risk of mediastinitis was small because, after division of the spur with the cricopharyngeus muscle in it, there was no longer any increase in pressure at the site of the lesion during deglutition. A residual diverticulum was found in 7% of the patients treated and Dohlman maintains that endoscopic treatment could always be repeated without difficulty in contrast to the problems which could be expected in a second external procedure.

Therapy

In Germany, Austria and England in particular, endoscopic treatment was widely used as demonstrated by the many publications from these countries since 1950.

Legler (1952), published his first report on 93 patients with a hypopharyngeal diverticulum treated endoscopically. Legler was a staunch advocate of this procedure, but pointed out that it should be carried out only by experienced hands. The complications reported in the literature, he believed, are to be regarded as a warning against any general recommendation of endoscopic treatment. He maintained that endoscopic treatment, which involved division of the cricopharyngeus muscle, eliminated the cause of the diverticulum. Prior to this treatment, passage of diverticular content into the oesophagus was only possible during swallowing, when the cricopharyngeus muscle relaxed. After division, overflow into the oesophagus was also possible without deglutition. Legler divided the septum down to the floor of the diverticulum with scissors without electrocoagulation, and he too regarded the risk of mediastinitis as small, in view of the possibility of adequate drainage via the wound and the use of antibiotics. He maintained that endoscopic treatment of small diverticula immediately eliminated dysphagia, and that after the treatment of medium-sized diverticula, connective tissue formation in the most distal part of the wound, could again lead to the formation of a low spur which he did not regard as a true recurrence. Repeated division was indicated in these cases and generally gave good results. Large diverticula also required several divisions, and in the presence of a very large diverticulum it could be necessary to excise a wedge-shaped part of the septum. None of the patients treated by Legler developed a haemorrhage, and he maintained that to prevent haemorrhage, it was strictly necessary to remain in the midline and particular caution was required in dealing with patients who had undergone previous surgery in the same site. Legler (1972), reported on 196 patients treated during the period 1948–1971. A complete cure as obtained by one or several divisions was obtained in 193 of these patients. Postoperative symptoms of mediastinitis (pyrexia, pain in the chest and between the shoulder blades) developed in 10 patients, and radiological examination showed subcutaneous and mediastinal emphysema. The mediastinal reaction in these patients responded well to conservative treatment. Three patients died in the postoperative period. In one case this was due to the blind introduction of a probe on the 5th postoperative day, which proved to have passed into the mediastinum. The second patient died as a result of bronchopneumonia, and the third from a pulmonary embolism.

Several authors (Paulsen and Keil, 1970; Juby, 1969 and Holinger, 1969) maintain that endoscopic treatment is to be regarded as the

Micro-endoscopic CO_2 laser surgery

treatment of choice in elderly patients whose general condition is poor. It appears that risk of haemorrhage in endoscopic treatment is small, and this is supported by the scarcity of reports of this complication in the literature. Lewis and Edwards (1962), described seven patients treated endoscopically with electrocoagulation, in one of whom a haemorrhage occurred. They did not attempt to arrest this endoscopically, but immediately undertook exploration of the neck. Todd (1974), mentioned some 'troublesome haemorrhage' in a total of 75 endoscopic treatments carried out in 58 patients in the manner described by Dohlman. Although the first endoscopic treatments were carried out in the USA (Mosher, Boston), the scanty American literature indicates that this method has not become very popular in that country. Holinger (1969), widely experienced in the treatment of hypopharyngeal diverticula, used both one-stage diverticulectomy and endoscopic treatment according to Dohlman. He mentioned that residual diverticula after division cause few symptoms and in no case did he observe enlargement of residual diverticula over the course of time. If a residual diverticulum after endoscopic treatment did cause symptoms he maintained that repeated endoscopic treatment was always possible. Holinger and also Harrison (1958), maintained that endoscopic treatment was to be preferred for elderly patients.

Trible (1975), after having treated 25 patients endoscopically with favourable results and without complications, listed brevity of the operation, low morbidity, and no recurrent laryngeal nerve damage, as advantages of this procedure.

6.2.3 PATIENTS AND METHODS

The ENT Department of the Groningen University Hospital, the Netherlands, has treated Zenker's diverticulum endoscopically since 1964. From then until 1986 413 patients with a diverticulum were admitted to our clinic and except for one of the two patients with a carcinoma of the pouch all were treated endoscopically, and no patient was refused surgery. Ten of the patients were suffering from a recurrent diverticulum after previous surgical diverticulectomy elsewhere.

We began to treat Zenker's diverticulum endoscopically, using the procedure described by Dohlman (1960), and we continue to believe in the advantages of endoscopic treatment and the good results that can be obtained with it (Overbeek and Hoeksema, 1982).

With the increase in the number of patients the technique and instruments used have been improved (Overbeek, Hoeksema and Edens, 1984). In 1981 we began to apply a micro-endoscopic procedure with a specially designed 'scope (Figure 6.1) and the operating micro-

Therapy

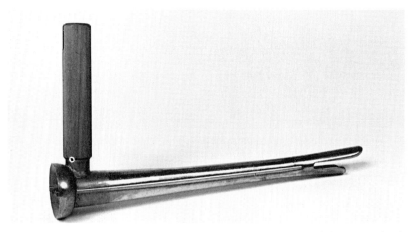

Figure 6.1 Lateral view of the scope applied for severance of the tissue bridge between oesophagus and diverticulum under microscopic control.

scope. The 'scope, with a total length of 25 cm, has a divided end with light channels in both lateral walls. Once the 'scope has been adjusted and fixed with a chest support, the light fibres are replaced by cannulae for continuous suction. These are necessary to remove the smoke of electrocoagulation and the steam, with its disagreeable odour associated with the use of the CO_2 laser.

To facilitate location of the oesophageal inlet during endoscopy, the patient is asked to swallow a black thread with a small metallic pellet at the end on the evening before endoscopic treatment. Before the operation, radiofluoroscopy is carried out in order to locate the pellet, and even when the pellet lies in the diverticulum, the thread can still be a useful aid in locating the oesophageal inlet, for in such cases oesophagoscopy often discloses that a loop of thread lies in the inlet.

Although endoscopic skill is required, exposure of the tissue bridge with the aid of the 'scope generally poses no special problems. Once the longer, upper lip of the 'scope is in position behind the arytenoids, the larynx is lifted and at the same time the 'scope is advanced, and in many cases the upper lip enters the oesophageal inlet almost automatically. The shorter lip finds its way into the lumen of the diverticulum without any difficulty, and the tissue bridge is caught – as it were – between the two lips, and once the spur is in focus, the chest support is attached to the 'scope. In order to avoid restriction to respiration, the chest support is rested on a table lying over the patient (Figure 6.2). The operating microscope with a conventional 400 mm objective affords a splendid view of the bridge to be divided (Figure 6.3A). For the technique of

Micro-endoscopic CO_2 laser surgery

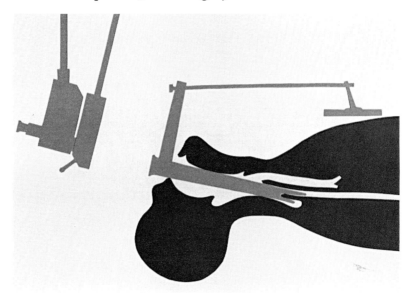

Figure 6.2 Diagram showing the scope in position and the CO_2 laser micromanipulator coupled with the operating microscope.

micro-endoscopic surgery, a general anaesthetic is necessary, but when there is a contraindication to a general anaesthetic from the patient's general condition, endoscopic treatment may be performed under local anaesthesia with the oesophagoscope and an electrocoagulation technique.

In micro-endoscopic surgery, very precise division of the tissue bridge between oesophagus and diverticulum is possible, either by electrocoagulation using insulated microsurgical instruments, or with the CO_2 laser (Overbeek, Hoeksema and Edens, 1984). Initially we feared that emphysema and mediastinitis would be more frequently found but the frequency of these complications is no different with the two techniques, and with both the wound edges separate immediately resulting in a wedged-shaped excision (Figure 6.3B). This separation is caused by retraction of the severed cricopharyngeus muscle fibres, which are readily identifiable through the microscope. In recent years we have used the CO_2 laser in nearly all patients, as we believe that the laser causes less tissue necrosis, and should therefore, produce less fibrous scar tissue.

A Sharplan CO_2 laser (35 W) has been used to divide the tissue bridge with wet gauze to protect the oesophagus and diverticulum. With the CO_2 laser the procedure sometimes produces slightly more bleeding

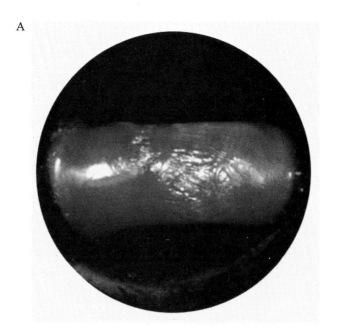

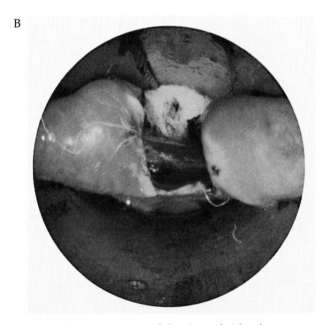

Figure 6.3 Micro-endoscopic views of the tissue bridge between oesophagus and diverticulum. (A) Before treatment; (B) After severance with the CO_2 laser.

Micro-endoscopic CO_2 laser surgery

than has usually been experienced with electrocoagulation, and when the bleeding is too severe to be controlled with the laser, brief electrocoagulation using an insulated microsurgical forcep or insulated suction tube can achieve haemostasis. It has been our impression that patients treated with the CO_2 laser suffered less pain during the first postoperative day, and consequently took food more readily. After the operation all patients were given antibiotics and liquid food for one week.

In patients with very large diverticula, we preferred to divide the spur in two or three sessions, guided by barium swallow radiographs and the patient's symptoms. In some cases there is radiological evidence of a residual diverticulum, but these patients are usually quite free from symptoms. Repetition of endoscopic treatment is always possible, but a small residual spur is not treated further unless the patient has residual symptoms (Figure 6.4). Although diagnostic radiology is indispensable in the postoperative phase and during the follow-up period, the information obtained from it should not be overestimated, and the patient's subjective well-being is at least as important as a criterion of successful treatment.

6.2.4 RESULTS

For the 377 patients treated endoscopically between 1964 and 1984, the follow-up is at least one year, and we believe that none of these patients has since been treated elsewhere. Of the 377 patients, 339 (90%) are highly satisfied and 36 (9.5%) are fairly satisfied with the results obtained. Although one patient died two days postoperatively from cardiac failure, the complications we observed were mostly not serious and the rate of complications was very low (Table 6.1).

The risk of mediastinitis is small suggesting the presence of adhesions between the diverticulum and the posterior oesophageal wall. Radiological follow-up revealed no essential difference in the final results between the patients treated with the electrocoagulation technique or with the CO_2 laser. In our laser patients, however, we have not noticed a tendency to stenosis, which has been seen in eight patients treated with electrocoagulation.

6.3 Discussion

The results which we have obtained in endoscopic treatment of the hypopharyngeal diverticulum prompted us to continue and further perfect this technique throughout the years, and it is somewhat surpris-

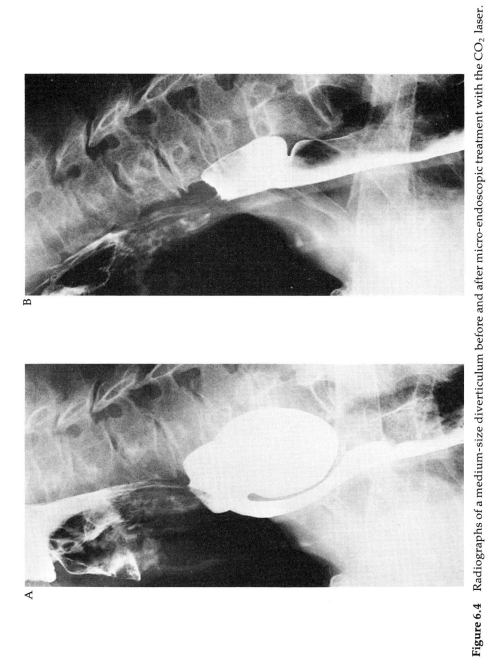

Figure 6.4 Radiographs of a medium-size diverticulum before and after micro-endoscopic treatment with the CO_2 laser.

Micro-endoscopic CO_2 laser surgery

Table 6.1 Complications after endoscopic treatment of hypopharyngeal diverticulum in 377 patients. (Combinations in 3 patients, follow-up at least one year.)

	Electrocoagulation *308 patients*	*CO_2 laser* *69 patients*
Mortality	1 – two days postoperative by cardiac failure	0
Mediastinitis	5 – cured by conservative therapy	3 – mediastinotomy 1 patient
Haemorrhage	4 – endoscopically controlled by coagulation	1 – stopped by tamponage
Oesophagotracheal fistula	1 – closed spontaneously within three weeks	0
Tendency to stenosis	8 – endoscopic dilations gave satisfactory results	0

ing that endoscopic treatment of Zenker's diverticulum has not become more popular. An important advantage of endoscopic treatment is that it can be carried out in patients whose general condition is poor, and although the procedure requires experience, we believe that experience is also important in diverticulectomy by an external approach.

Exposure of the tissue bridge between the oesophagus and diverticulum with the aid of the specially designed 'scope with a divided end, and facilities for fixation, pose no significant problems. The use of the operating microscope is found to be a great improvement in the endoscopic treatment, and very precise severance of the spur is possible with the aid of insulated microsurgical instruments or a CO_2 laser. The magnification makes it possible to identify the nature of the tissues in the plane of division and to follow the separation of the muscle fibres. Haemorrhage, when it occurs, can be arrested without causing more than minimal damage.

From the good results that we have obtained, it can be stated that the micro-endoscopic technique with the CO_2 laser is an improvement on the original Dohlman's method.

References

Dohlman, G. (1949), Endoscopic operations for hypopharyngeal diverticula. *Proc. 4e Int. Congr. Otolaryngol. London*, 715–17.

Dohlman, G. and Mattsson, O. (1960), The endoscopic operation for hypopharyngeal diverticula. *Arch. Otolaryngol*, **71**, 744–52.

References

Ellis, F. H., Schlegel, J. F., Lynch, V. P. and Payne, W. S. (1969), Cricopharyngeal myotomy for pharyngo-esophageal diverticulum, *Ann. Surg.*, **170**, 340–50.

Harrison, M. S. (1958), The aetiology, diagnosis and surgical treatment of pharyngeal diverticula. *J. Laryngol. Otol.*, **72**, 523–34.

Holinger, P. H. and Schild, J. A. (1969), The Zenker's (hypopharyngeal) diverticulum. *Ann. Otol. Rhinol. Laryngol.*, **78**, 679–88.

Juby, H. B. (1969), The treatment of pharyngeal pouch. *J. Laryngol. Otol.*, **83**, 1067–71.

Killian, G. (1908), Ueber den Mund der Speizeröhre. *Zeitschr. Ohrenheilkd und Krankheiten Luftwege*, **55**, 1–41.

Lahey, F. H. and Warren, K. W. (1954), Esophageal diverticula. *Surg. Gynecol. Obstet.*, **98**, 1–28.

Legler, U. (1952), Untersuchungen vor und nach endoskopischer Operation kleiner und grosser Hypopharynxdivertikel. *Arch. Klin. Exp. Ohren. Nasen. Kehlkopfheilkd*, **160**, 547–60.

Legler, U. (1972), Le traitement endoscopique du diverticule oesophagopharyngien (Zenker). *J. Fr. Otorhinolaryngol.*, **21**, 775–90.

Lewis, R. S. and Edwards, W. G. (1962), The treatment of pharyngeal diverticula. *Br. J. Surg.*, **50**, 1–5.

Mosher, H. P. (1917), Webs and pouches of the oesophagus, their diagnosis and treatment. *Surg. Gynecol. Obstet.*, **25**, 175–87.

Mosher, H. P. (1929), *The nose, throat and ear and their diseases*. C. Jackson, G. M. Coates, W. B. Saunders Comp., Philadelphia and London, pp. 1055–62.

Mosher, H. P. (1935), The oesophagus. *Surg. Gynecol. Obstet.*, **60**, 403–17.

Overbeek, J. J. M. van. (1977), The hypopharyngeal diverticulum. *Endoscopic treatment and manometry*. Van Gorcum, Assen, the Netherlands.

Overbeek, J. J. M. van and Hoeksema, P. E. (1982) Endoscopic treatment of the hypopharyngeal diverticulum: 211 cases. *Laryngoscope*, **92**, 88–91.

Overbeek, J. J. M. van, Hoeksema, P. E. and Edens, E. Th. (1984), Microendoscopic surgery of the hypopharyngeal diverticulum using electrocoagulation or carbon dioxide laser. *Ann. Otol. Rhinol. Laryngol.*, **93**, 34–6.

Paulsen, K. and Keil, H. (1970), Komplikationshäufigkeit und Rezidivquote nach endoskopischer Schwellenspaltung des Zenkerschen Divertikels. *Monatschr. Ohrenheilkd. Laryngorhinol.*, **109**, 554–60.

Schubel, J. (1947), Beitrag zur operativen Behandlung der Hypopharynxdivertikel vom Hypopharynxlumen aus. *Zentralbl. Chir.*, **9**, 941–6.

Seiffert, A. (1932), Zur Behandlung beginnender Hypopharyngdivertikel. *Z. Laryngol. Rhinol. Laryngol.*, **23**, 256–8.

Serles, W. (1967), Ueber die Behandlung des Zenkerschen Hypopharynxdivertikels. *Monatschr. Ohrenheilkd. Laryngorhinol.*, **101**, 401–8.

Todd, G. B. (1974), The treatment of pharyngeal pouch. *J. Laryngol. Otol.*, **88**, 307–15.

Trible, W. M. (1975), The surgical treatment of Zenker's diverticulum: Endoscopic vs external operation. *South. Med. J.*, **68**, 1260–2.

7 The role of lasers in nasal surgery

A. P. BRIGHTWELL

Since the development of the continuous wave CO_2 laser in 1962, its role in a wide range of surgical disciplines has been extensively researched. The CO_2 laser is now a well established tool in ENT for the management of a wide range of benign and malignant lesions, particularly within the oral cavity and larynx. The first report of the use of lasers in rhinology was by Lenz in 1977 who described inferior turbinectomy using the argon laser in patients with vasomotor rhinitis. He found the main advantages to be excellent haemostasis and minimal patient discomfort, although the availability and cost of equipment was seen to be a major problem. A variety of reports have followed this including Simpson, Shapshay and Vaughan (1983) who detailed the use of the CO_2 laser in 42 patients with a wide range of nasal conditions over a period of 10 years.

However, when treating common nasal problems, in order for laser surgery to be widely accepted, and for its costs and hazards to be justified, it has to be shown to have significant advantages over established, conventional techniques. Undoubtedly, in patients suffering from bleeding disorders or in those with particularly haemorrhagic lesions, the excellent haemostatic properties may make the laser the treatment of choice.

Three lasers, the CO_2, argon and Nd-YAG are most widely used in clinical practice and of these, most of the work has been carried out with the CO_2 and argon lasers, but it appears that the Nd-YAG laser may prove to be of value in this field in the future.

7.1 The CO_2 laser

The advantages of the CO_2 laser are related to its absorption and method of tissue destruction. The far infrared beam is absorbed by water and tissue removal is by instantaneous vaporization at the

The role of lasers in nasal surgery

relatively low temperature of 100°C. This results in high precision cutting with minimal thermal damage to adjacent, normal tissues, particularly when high laser power densities are used. Postoperative oedema and scar tissue formation are minimal and this may lead to a reduction in adhesion formation within the nasal cavity. The CO_2 laser also provides good haemostasis for most lesions as it coagulates vessels of up to 0.5 mm in diameter, resulting in a relatively bloodless field and a reduced need for postoperative nasal packing which many patients find particularly unpleasant. This property of the CO_2 laser is of particular relevance when operating on patients with bleeding disorders. Other well-documented advantages include minimal postoperative discomfort, rapid wound healing and reduced instrumentation and manipulation of tissues.

The CO_2 laser is a cutting instrument and can be used either to excise or vaporize lesions. It is most useful when treating conditions of the mucous membranes rather than skin, but extra care has to be taken when operating on nasal mucosa adjacent to cartilage. Williams and Mitchell (1980) in histological studies using rabbits whose nasal mucosa and septum are comparable to humans, have shown that repair of keratinized mucosa occurs rapidly within seven days of lasering, although respiratory epithelium heals more slowly. The nasal septum, however, was shown to be vulnerable to lasering and more than three exposures of 100 ms duration at a power of 4 W to the mucosa caused underlying cartilage necrosis which was then replaced by fibrous tissue despite normal epithelial healing. This limitation is particularly important when treating bilateral lesions of the nasal septum. Vaporization of bone is not practical as the temperature of destruction for this non-water containing tissue is extremely high. This results in both slower and poorer healing with increased thermal damage to adjacent tissues.

The short-term results of patients treated with this laser appear encouraging, but to date there have been no controlled trials to compare the long-term results of laser surgery with those achieved by conventional techniques. It is hoped particularly that adhesion formation and nasal stenosis should be reduced and there is a theoretical advantage of reduced tumour dissemination by lymphatics which are sealed by the laser beam.

7.2 The argon laser

The argon laser is selectively absorbed by red pigments and it can be used to seal vessels of up to 1 mm in diameter. Its greatest value in rhinology is in the treatment of vascular abnormalities where, at low power settings, it will obliterate submucosal vessels with minimal

Laser technique

damage to the overlying normal mucosa. At higher power levels vaporization of tissue can be performed.

Lenz (1980) described a series of 308 patients on whom he performed endonasal surgery, mostly for treatment of hypertrophied inferior turbinates in vasomotor rhinitis. Using the argon laser, excellent haemostasis was found with minimal patient discomfort. An *in vitro* study has shown that it is technically possible to cut bone to form intra-nasal antrostomies, at a power setting of 20 W with a beam diameter of 0.1 mm, although the author points out that a flexible guiding system would have to be developed for clinical use (Lenz *et al.*, 1977). Furthermore, it has been shown that a larger extent of tissue necrosis is caused than is evident at the time of surgery as a result of vascular occlusion at the edge of the excision. With the limited availability and versatility of argon lasers their main indication for use at present is in the treatment of vascular conditions, and in particular, hereditary haemorrhagic telangectasia.

7.3 The Nd-YAG laser

The Nd-YAG laser is the most powerful continuous wave laser producing low infrared coherent light, which is deeply absorbed in the tissues without colour or tissue specificity. The deep absorption means that when used to carry out thermal tissue destruction, a large overall volume of tissue is removed and blood vessels of up to 1.5 mm in diameter may be sealed. The beam can be delivered by a flexible fibreoptic system which allows treatment of lesions in areas which are inaccessible to the rigid endoscope which is necessary with the CO_2 laser. Although its use has been described in the treatment of hereditary haemorrhagic telangectasia (Parkin and Dixon, 1981), there is at present no accepted role for the Nd-YAG laser in rhinology, although it has been used to a limited extent in other otolaryngological conditions. Its value in the thermal removal of tumour tissue has been clearly demonstrated in the treatment of inoperable tumour obstructing both the oesophagus and tracheobronchial tree.

7.4 Laser technique

The CO_2 laser is mounted on an operating microscope with both the focal point of the laser and of the lens at 300 mm. This provides excellent illumination and magnification of the operative field, and the beam is positioned with great accuracy with a micromanipulator aiming sys-

The role of lasers in nasal surgery

tem. Anterior lesions of the nasal cavity are readily accessible with the aid of any conventional speculum. Alternatively a large aural speculum with a self-supporting holder, frees one of the surgeon's hands and also provides protection of the alar margin (Figure 7.1). However, it should be remembered that although these anodized instruments do not reflect the microscope light, the infrared laser beam is still reflected almost as effectively as by a shiny metal surface. The surrounding areas of the face are further protected against accidental exposure to the laser beam by a wet, thick, gauze swab placed around the speculum (Figure 7.2). A non-combustible, metal sucker must also be used at all times, to remove the steam produced by tissue vaporization, both to allow visual access and to prevent thermal damage of the tissues by the steam.

The majority of lesions within the nasal cavity can be vaporized without submitting the specimen to histological examination. In comparison to other sites, excision of nasal lesions is more difficult but can be performed on anterior septal lesions. When operating on more posteriorly placed lesions, a wet gauze swab should be placed in the post-nasal space to provide both a landmark and protection of the Eustachian tube orifices. Access to the post-nasal space itself is

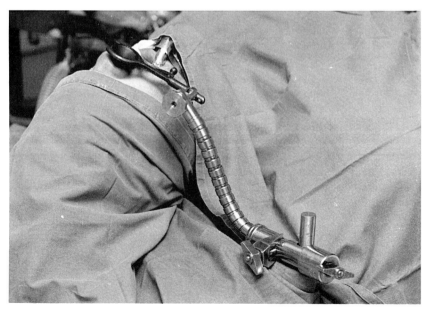

Figure 7.1 The use of an aural speculum and holder to provide access to the anterior nasal space with protection of the alar margin.

Laser technique

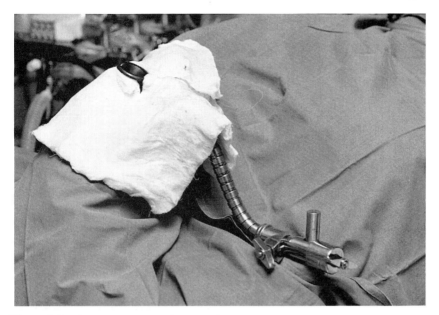

Figure 7.2 A wet gauze swab provides extra protection to the surrounding facial skin against accidental laser irradiation.

achieved with the patient in the tonsil position, and using stainless-steel mirrors to reflect the laser beam behind the soft palate. Only metal instruments should be used to retract the palate and suction can be provided either with a suction tube placed through the nasal cavity or by a yankeur sucker held by an assistant in the nasopharynx.

As with all CO_2 laser surgery the usual safety precautions must be taken to protect the patient, theatre staff and any combustible anaesthetic equipment. During endonasal surgery, the wet gauze in the nasopharynx will protect the anaesthetic tube, but when operating on the nasopharynx via the mouth, the anaesthetic tube should be either made of metal or wrapped with aluminium foil in the usual way.

The argon laser can be used either under local or general anaesthetic depending on both the retraction necessary for access and the amount of lasering anticipated. Delivery of the laser beam is most commonly via a handpiece which limits treatment to the external nose or to the anterior portion of the nasal cavity. All theatre staff must, of course, wear protective goggles and the patient's eyes are protected by either goggles or firmly fixed protective material such as adhesive aluminium tape.

The role of lasers in nasal surgery

7.5 Laser applications in the nose

7.5.1 THE EXTERNAL NOSE

The CO_2 laser is primarily an instrument for vaporization of mucosa rather than skin. Histological studies have shown that CO_2 incisions of skin heal more slowly, and at seven days have a lower tensile strength when compared with incisions cut by scalpel (Cochrane, 1980). However, in certain pathologies it is advantageous to use the CO_2 laser as a skin incising tool.

When treating rhinophyma by standard paring techniques, the two main problems encountered are excessive bleeding and difficulty in achieving smooth contours and demarcation with adjacent facial tissues. The excellent haemostasis achieved with the CO_2 laser enables bloodless ablation of the excess rhinophyma tissue to the required depth to be performed. This precise dissection facilitates the accurate sculpturing of the remaining nasal tissues to achieve a good cosmetic result. Shapshay *et al.* (1980) have described their early experience of this accurate and haemostatic technique, both under local and general anaesthetic. A standard excision of rhinophyma tissue is performed, leaving an intact rim of skin around the nares to prevent stenosis. Re-epithelialization occurs from the remnants of glandular epithelium with the initial formation of an eschar 24 h after surgery which remains for approximately ten days. Complete healing is achieved in the same time as with standard techniques, namely 3–4 weeks. No complications were reported and minimal patient discomfort and good to excellent cosmetic results were achieved in a majority of patients when assessed after six months.

A small series of patients with recurrent skin tumours to the external nose has been reported by Somma and Dioguardi (1982). These were excised with conventional margins using the CO_2 laser and the advantages of this method included a 'no touch' technique, a reduction in intra-operative bleeding which with the sealing of lymphatics might theoretically reduce the spread of tumour cells. However, improved cure rates have yet to be proven.

The argon laser can be used for the treatment of vascular lesions affecting the skin of the nose, such as telangectasia or port wine stains as well as the condition of post rhinoplasty red nose (Noe *et al.*, 1981). This is, happily, a rare complication usually of a revision procedure which results in a diffuse area of erythema and telangectasia on the dorsum of the nose. With the selective absorption of the argon laser beam by pigmented structures, vascular lesions may be successfully ablated without significant damage to the overlying epidermis.

Laser applications in the nose

7.5.2 THE ANTERIOR AND POSTERIOR NASAL SPACES

A wide range of lesions within the anterior nasal space can be treated effectively and safely using the CO_2 laser. Papillomas, granulomas, polyps and adhesions can all be excised or vaporized with great precision and minimal damage to adjacent, normal structures. In particular, partial removal of the anterior portion of hypertrophied inferior turbinates provides relief of nasal obstruction with a considerably reduced risk of bleeding, and in many cases nasal packing is unnecessary. Very selective, piecemeal vaporization of turbinate tissue is possible under excellent vision with preservation of the superior mucosal surface. Watery rhinorrhoea with nasal obstruction develops some six hours postoperatively, followed by the formation of crusts, with complete healing at 3–6 weeks. The end result is identical to conventional turbinectomy with regards to nasal obstruction, but most patients claim some additional symptomatic improvement from the symptoms of sneezing, nasal discharge and headaches (Mittleman, 1982).

Hereditary haemorrhagic telangectasia is a rare familial syndrome with abnormal, subepithelial, thin walled, vascular lesions causing frequent brisk epistaxes. The severity of this condition increases with age, presenting a difficult management problem. Conventional methods of treatment such as cautery, arterial embolization, septodermoplasty and oestrogen therapy have only limited success or can produce complications. Photocoagulation of lesions with the CO_2, argon or Nd-YAG laser can be performed, resulting in accurate and permanent obliteration of individual telangectatic spots without mucosal contact. Results so far have been promising with a reduction in both the severity and frequency of epistaxis and the need for blood transfusions. Regular, repeated treatments may be necessary as new telangectatic spots commonly develop in other areas and photocoagulation provides control of the symptoms rather than a cure for the disease.

The argon laser with its selective absorption by pigmented structures, is the most effective method for treating telangectasia leaving overlying mucosa intact and without causing damage to underlying cartilage or bone. The CO_2 laser can also be used to vaporize the nasal mucosa before obliterating the telangectasia and there is, of course, some slight risk of damage to the underlying septal cartilage, although good symptomatic control can be achieved using this laser. Better vascular control may be achieved with the Nd-YAG laser, but it may be that it should be reserved for the more extensive arteriovenous malformations which sometimes form in the more severe cases of hereditary haemorrhagic telangectasia.

More posteriorly placed lesions of the nasal cavity are less access-

The role of lasers in nasal surgery

ible, but choanal atresia in the neonate and child has been successfully treated using the CO_2 laser. An endonasal approach has been used with a wet gauze placed in the post-nasal space, both to identify when the atretic plate has been breached and also to protect the Eustachian tube orifices. In a series described by Healy et al. (1978) from Boston, ten sides were treated in patients aged 16 hours to 14 years, with seven remaining patent without further surgery. In two of the three failures, the technique was reperformed but only one remained patent. The operative advantages of this technique include accuracy, speed and haemostasis with reduced postoperative oedema and scarring which is particularly important in the neonatal airway. They also reported that the need for postoperative stenting could be reduced to 2–3 weeks. However, approximately 90% of all cases have a bony atretic plate and if it is thicker than 1 mm it should be removed by rongeur rather than laser, otherwise overheating of the surrounding bone and tissues may occur which could result in necrosis, sequestran and the formation of granulation and scar tissue.

Access to the post-nasal space can be achieved with the patient in the tonsil position and by reflecting the CO_2 laser beam into the nasopharynx with stainless-steel mirrors. This technique has been used in the Southampton Laser Unit to provide palliation for malignant tumours after radiotherapy failure and the possibility of control of smaller lesions exists.

7.5.3 THE PARANASAL SINUSES

A combination of limited access to the paranasal sinuses and the unsuitability of this technique for bone removal, results in reduced application for laser surgery in this field. Lenz (1977) has described how it is technically possible to cut antrostomies with the argon laser using *in vitro* specimens but admits that a guiding system would have to be developed for clinical use. Even with such a system positive advantages would have to be shown over conventional techniques in order to justify the cost.

Transantral, vidian neurectomy for vasomotor rhinitis using the CO_2 laser has been reported by Williams (1983) to have advantages over conventional surgical techniques. In this series the CO_2 laser was used to vaporize windows in both the thick anterior and thin posterior walls of the maxillary antrum without the complications due to overheating that might have been expected. The vidian canal was then identified in the pterygopalatine fossa, and its contents vaporized with a defocused beam which also produced haemostasis. When compared to conventional surgery the patients all reported less pain and oedema with reduced transient hyperaesthesia. The long-term results were found to be identical and the only complication reported in twelve patients was one epistaxis from an antrostomy fashioned conventionally.

Good control of recurrent, anterior skull based tumours can be achieved after failed surgery and radiotherapy. Tumours in the ethmoidal region can be excised or vaporized using the CO_2 laser with access via the maxillectomy cavity, provided that no intracranial spread is shown on CT scanning and polytomography. After removal of the macroscopic tumour, the bone of the skull base may be heated white hot to ensure that occult areas of tumour are destroyed. This avoids a major craniofacial resection and has a lower morbidity and may provide more effective palliation than chemotherapy. However, the overheating of bone can produce a CSF leak which might require plugging with a muscle graft. Some encouraging results have been reported by Rontal and Rontal (1983) in a small series of patients undergoing repeated lasering as necessary to palliate, and in some cases control this condition which previously had an extremely poor prognosis, both in terms of morbidity and mortality.

References

Cochrane, J. P. S., Deacon, J. P., Creasey, G. H. and Russell, R. C. G. (1980), Wound healing after laser surgery: an experimental study. *Br. J. Surg.*, **67**, 740.

Healy, G. B., McGill, T., Jako, G. J., Strong, M. S. and Vaughan, C. W. (1978), Management of choanal atresia with the Carbon Dioxide laser. *Ann. Otol. Rhinol. Laryngol.*, **87**, 658–62.

Lenz, H. (1980), Endonasal laser surgery. In *Lasers in Medicine* (ed. H. K. Koebner), Wiley, Chichester.

Lenz, H., Eichler, J., Schafer, G., Salk, J. and Bettges, G. (1977), Production of a nasoantral window with Ar laser. *J. Maxillofac. Surg.*, **5**, 314–7.

Mittleman, H. (1982), CO_2 laser turbinectomies for chronic obstructive rhinitis. *Lasers Surg. Med.*, **2**, 29–36.

Noe, J. M., Finley, J., Rosen, S. and Arndt, K. A. (1981), Post-rhiniplasty 'Red Nose': Differential diagnosis and treatment by laser. *Plast. Reconstr. Surg.*, **67**, 661–4.

Parkin, J. L. and Dixon, J. A. (1981), Laser photocoagulation in hereditary haemorrhagic telangectasia. *Otolaryngol. Head Neck Surg.*, **89**, 204–8.

Rontal, M. and Rontal, E. (1983), Treatment of recurrent carcinoma at the base of the skull with carbon dioxide laser. *Laryngoscope*, **93**, 1261–5.

Shapshay, S. M., Strong, M. S., Anastasi, G. W. and Vaughan, C. W. (1980), Removal of rhinophyma with the carbon dioxide laser: A preliminary report. *Arch. Otolaryngol.*, **106**, 257–9.

Simpson, G. T., Shapshay, S. M. and Vaughan, C. W. (1983), Rhinological laser surgery. *Otolaryngol. Clin. North Am.*, **16**, 829–37.

The role of lasers in nasal surgery

Somma, A. M. and Dioguardi, D. (1982), CO_2 laser surgery in recurrent tumours of the nose. *Am. Plast. Surg.*, **9**, 172–4.

Williams, D. J. and Mitchell, D. P. (1980), The laser and the nasal septum – a histological study. *J. Otolaryngol.*, **9**, 12–17.

Williams, J. D. (1983), Laser vidian neurectomy. *Ann. Otol. Rhinol. Laryngol.*, **92**, 281–3.

8 The use of the laser in otology

J. J. PHILLIPPS

The use of the laser in ENT surgery has for the most part been confined to surgery of the oral cavity and the larynx. The benefits that the laser confers in these areas are now well accepted: the precise bloodless dissection which it allows, the clear view obtained down an operating microscope, since there is only minimal instrumentation, and lastly the fact that only minimal damage is done to the tissues which surround the area that has been treated. In middle ear surgery, the ideal conditions are those of a bloodless field, where one has a clear view of the pathology involved – combined with surgical skills which allow one to manipulate one's instruments in an exacting fashion. It might seem from the above that the surgical laser was designed with the middle ear in mind, yet at the present time lasers are used relatively rarely in otology and little has been written about the use of the laser in this field. The main reason why otologists have been slow to take up the laser is the fear that its use in the middle ear might have serious sequelae – in particular the possibility of damage to the inner ear. In addition to this, before there will be widespread use of the laser, it will be necessary to demonstrate that its use is not only safe, but also that the results which are obtained with it are better than those achieved with conventional methods; only this would justify the considerable expenditure which is inevitably involved.

8.1 Experimental background

There have been two main areas of research: first the effects of the laser irradiation upon the inner ear, and secondly the more specific effects of the laser when used in the region of the footplate.

The first assessment of the effect of the laser upon the inner ear was reported by Stahle and Hogberg in 1965. Using a ruby laser the lateral canals of pigeons were irradiated. Histological examination of the lasered areas showed atrophy of the epithelium of the inner ear together with a marked fibrous reaction. The damage was assumed to be mainly due to a thermal effect, but it was thought that there was a possible secondary effect due to ultrasonic vibration.

Kelemen, Laor and Klein (1967), gave high doses of pulsed irradiation to the heads of mice using ruby and neodymium lasers. The exposed sites included the forehead, the intact region of the external ear, and surgically exposed sites on the skull and brain. They found that animals treated in the same way showed damage or lack of it on an 'all or none' response. When damage to the inner ear did occur, it was found that the vestibular end organ was more vulnerable than the cochlea. This damage to the inner ear was present when the ear itself had not been directly exposed to the laser. Skin and bone were often relatively uninjured whilst there was a deeper secondary effect. These intracranial lesions were thought to be produced by transmission of pressure, or possibly a shock wave as a result of the interactions of the tissues. A similar warning of secondary effects of laser irradiation was given by Fox (1968), who found that pulses of high energy laser irradiation to the skull could explode the enclosed structures because of over-pressurization caused by vaporization of the underlying tissues. Such intracranial explosion did not occur if continuous wave irradiation was used.

Stahle, Hogberg and Engstrom (1972) using the argon laser focused the beam directly onto the cochlea of guinea pigs. This caused an immediate burn to the mucous membrane, but at no time was the otic capsule penetrated by the laser beam. However, upon opening the bony capsule of the cochlea, an obvious tissue reaction was found on the stria vascularis adjacent to the point of impact on the otic capsule. The damage in the cochlea was confined to this area alone.

Wilpizeski *et al.* (1972) used an argon continuous wave laser to irradiate the lateral semicircular canals of squirrel monkeys, in some cases sufficiently to penetrate the bony wall. Pre-operatively the monkeys had had vestibular assessments using caloric and body rotation tests. Two of the monkeys had been trained to track their auditory thresholds by a conditioned avoidance response procedure. Animals with non-penetrating irradiation showed little change in their vestibular function except for slight ataxia for the first postoperative day, and only slight reduction in the caloric response. The body rotation tests were unchanged. Animals which had a penetrating injury were found to have a marked fibrous reaction within the membranous labyrinth. They suffered from ataxia and poor acrobatic ability, and there was a reduction in the response to caloric stimulation. The hearing acuity of the two trained animals remained within normal limits, even though there was obvious vestibular dysfunction. Wilpizeski *et al.* conclude by stating 'serious consideration should be given by otologists to the experimental evaluation of lasers for human purposes', and they suggest such applications as myringotomy, footplate removal, ossicle amputation and cochlear lesions.

The first assessment of the effects of the laser specifically on the stapes footplate was reported by Sataloff in 1967. He used a neodymium laser on normal and otoscleratic footplates *in vitro*. The neodymium laser is not absorbed by white or non-pigmented tissue, and by itself had no effect upon the foot plate unless the tissue surface was pigmented artificially. Copper sulphate (which is toxic to the human ear), was used to allow the absorbtion of laser energy onto the footplate. It was possible to produce discrete lesion in the footplate, but a warning was made about the possibility of transmission of energy to deeper levels with subsequent damage.

There are few further experimental studies on the effect of laser energy on the footplate until Perkins reported the first clinical trial of laser stapedotomy in 1980. Prior to carrying out his operations *in vivo*, he assessed the effect of the argon laser in post-mortem temporal bones. These were used to evaluate the parameters of the laser beam necessary to vaporize small holes in the footplate. Subsequently the footplate was removed and the macculae of the saccule and the adjacent medial vestibular wall were inspected through the operating microscope for evidence of damage. No damage was found, but no formal histological assessment was carried out. A very similar assessment was carried out by Di Bartolomeo (1980); again the footplate was fenestrated and then removed and the vestibule 'examined for any adventitious changes'. No histology was performed.

Following on from Perkins and Di Bartolomeo's experimental work and subsequent clinical trials, Gantz *et al.* (1982) carried out a histological investigation of the changes in the middle ear and vestibule following argon laser fenestration of the stapes footplate in cats. A rosette pattern of small fenestra was created on the footplate and the central portion was vaporized usually with a single pulse – care being taken not to pass the beam directly through the fenestration. Light microscopy of the specimens was then performed. In three of eight ears a perforation in the saccular membrane was found in direct line with the laser fenestration of the footplate. The authors noted that in footplates with less pigmentation, more pulses of energy were required to produce a char, and that although the pulse duration was only of 0.1 s, the final portion of bone might be vaporized at the beginning of the pulse allowing the beam to penetrate more deeply. Since the argon laser passes through clear fluids, the beam would continue until meeting a pigmented structure – the saccule.

An investigation of the thermal effects of argon laser fenestration of

The use of the laser in otology

the footplate was reported by Ricci and Mazzoni (1985). A thermocouple was placed in the vestibule, and then the footplate was perforated using the laser. They were only able to demonstrate a small temperature increment and concluded that the argon laser could be used with confidence during stapedectomy or tympanoplasty. However, other investigators were less confident. Thoma (1981) showed that apart from thermal reactions as a consequence of laser irradiation to the footplate, endocochlear pressure fluctuations may also cause functional damage to the inner ear. In 1986, Thoma, Mrowinski and Kastenbauer assessed the suitability of the CO_2 laser as an alternative to the argon laser for stapedotomy. In the normal footplate it was found that the CO_2 laser caused less thermal stress than the argon laser, but when a perforation was induced in a thickened footplate, then the change in temperature and pressure was so great that functional damage to the cochlea could not be precluded. The CO_2 laser was thought to be unsuitable for use in otosclerotic ears.

8.2 Clinical applications

In the field of otology, both the argon and the CO_2 lasers have been employed. The two lasers have different qualities, but in particular the argon laser has a greater ability to coagulate vessels, and has the advantage (in middle ear surgery), of being able to obtain smaller spot sizes than the CO_2 laser. In both cases the laser is mounted onto the operating microscope, and the site where the laser beam will strike is demonstrated by an aiming beam. The beam is manoeuvred by a micromanipulator. As in any other field of laser surgery, strict safety precautions are always followed (see Chapter 1).

8.3 External ear and external auditory meatus

There would appear to be no specific otological indications for the use of lasers on the pinna, although dermatological conditions such as port wine stains may be treated with the argon laser. There is a report of the argon laser being used to excise pedunculated osteomas of the ear canal (Di Bartolomeo, 1980) but this would not appear to have any real advantage over conventional methods. The CO_2 laser could be used to excise areas of meatal stenosis, but there would always be the worry of potential damage to the underlying tissues.

Tympanic membrane and middle ear

8.4 Tympanic membrane and middle ear

8.4.1 MYRINGOTOMY

In the treatment of patients with secretory otitis media, a decision needs to be made whether to treat the condition with myringotomy alone or whether to insert a grommet. If a myringotomy alone is performed then the drum may heal within 2–3 days, which may be insufficient to allow the mucosal changes in the middle ear to resolve. On the other hand, if a grommet is inserted, this may stay in place for an excessive period of time, may be associated with scarring of the drum, and many surgeons will still advise avoidance of swimming whilst the grommets are in place – a source of much distress to many children. It has been suggested that by using a laser to perform myringotomies, this might allow the myringotomy to remain open for a period of three to four weeks and thus to allow the vicious circle to be broken.

Goode (1982) reported the use of the CO_2 laser to perform myringotomies in 12 ears. He was able to produce a 2 mm perforation using a single 0.1 s pulse. His patients were untypical of secretory otitis media in that four patients had middle ear effusions secondary to head and neck cancer procedures and/or radiation to the nasopharynx. Only three of the 10 patients were under the age of 5 years. Two out of the twelve myringotomies failed to heal; one where the perforation had been made in a monomeric membrane, and another where a 4 mm hole had been deliberately made to try to make a permanent perforation in a patient with hyperpatent Eustachian tube. Of those that did heal, the perforation had closed within six weeks. It was emphasized that to perform myringotomies in an ear without an effusion would lead to a burn on the promontory, and in such cases it would be necessary to inject saline into the middle ear prior to the myringotomy. A larger series of patients was reported by Lipman *et al.* (1987); 100 patients, who would otherwise have had grommets inserted, underwent myringotomies using the CO_2 laser. No details of the ages of the patients are given, nor any analysis of the aetiology of the middle ear effusions. The laser myringotomies remained open for 2–4 weeks, and only 40% developed recurrent effusions, although there was no control group of patients who had incisional myringotomy alone. No comment was made whether any perforations failed to heal. Both sets of authors emphasize that the procedure could be performed under local iontophoretic anaesthesia, thus potentially cutting the costs of the operation, although Goode admits the difficulty of getting sufficient co-operation in young children, who, of course, comprise the majority of patients requiring such surgery.

The use of the laser in otology

Laser myringotomy will be a safe procedure in the majority of cases, although it should be avoided in the atelectatic drum, or if there is suspicion that the drum is retracted down onto the promontory. Similarly it must be avoided in cases where there is no middle ear effusion (not necessarily an easy thing to establish until a myringotomy has been performed), or burns to the medial wall of the middle ear will occur. The possible benefits are that it may mean the avoidance of grommets, but it is unclear from the reports so far what percentage of patients would benefit since no control group has been used.

8.4.2 TYMPANOPLASTY

The first clinical report of the use of the laser in otology came from Escudero *et al.* (1979). In a series of seven myringoplasties the argon laser was used initially to coagulate small vessels in the external canal and on the tympanic membrane, and when the temporalis fascia graft had been placed onto the drum remnant as an onlay, the graft was then 'spot-welded' to the underlying cone of the external canal. Precise postoperative details are not given, in particular no length of follow up is stated, but no rejection of any form was recorded. Di Bartolomeo used a similar technique in a further series of seven patients. He noted a tendency for the laser to cause some immediate shrinkage of the graft, but this problem was overcome by having a graft which was not stretched to its maximum limit. Six of his seven cases were successful; one patient having a small residual defect which was eventually closed with 'office stimulation'. The same author suggested that the laser could be used to divide middle ear adhesions, and also to 'sculpture' ossicles for replacement in the middle ear.

The papers referred to above concern only very small series and although they show that the laser may be used without any apparent problems, they fail to demonstrate any clear advantage over conventional techniques.

8.4.3 CHRONIC SUPPURATIVE OTITIS MEDIA

It is in inflammatory conditions of the middle ear cleft that one finds some situations where the laser may actually have some advantages over conventional techniques. In spite of hypotensive anaesthetics and local infiltration of vasoconstrictors, mastoid surgery may still be quite bloody, and the coagulating qualities of the argon laser may be useful. Palva suggests that the laser may be useful in removing disease atraumatically from the stapes footplate. McGee (1983) considers the three ways in which the laser can alter tissue: by vaporizing, cutting and coagulating. Using a spot size of 1–2 mm at an output of 1.8–2 W for 0.1–0.2 s he used it safely in the middle ear to vaporize granulations, scar tissue, pigmented cholesteatomas and mucosal bands. If it was necessary to vaporize tissues in the area of the oval or round windows then the spot size was reduced as was the power output. He used the laser as a cutting tool to remove dense scar tissue in cases of revision mastoid surgery, and found it to be quicker and much less bloody than using conventional methods. The laser was effective as a coagulator of small vessels around the oval window and on the promontory, and was also used successfully and safely to stop micro bleeding on the facial nerve during three facial nerve decompressions.

8.4.4 OTOSCLEROSIS

In the operation of stapedectomy, if the removal or fenestration of the footplate is performed traumatically then a severe sensorineural hearing loss may ensue. The laser offers the possibility of working on the footplate whilst ensuring that no movement will take place, potentially a great advantage providing no undesirable side effects occur. Perkins (1980) performed a laser stapedotomy in eleven patients using the argon laser to vaporize the stapedius tendon and the posterior crus, together with the anterior crus if this was visible. Having exposed the footplate, multiple small holes were made in the footplate in a rosette fashion, using a small spot size and a power output of 0.4–0.7 W for 0.1 s thus creating a small bone disc which was removed using a 45° pick, leaving behind a stapedotomy fenestra. The stapedectomy was then completed in the usual way. Although his postoperative follow up was rather short, in no patient was the postoperative bone conduction less than it had been pre-operatively. All patients had closure of the air-bone gap between 0 and 10 db.

McGee (1983) reported on a much larger series of stapedectomies, comparing the results of patients who had a laser stapedotomy with those who had a small window fenestra using conventional techniques. Like Perkins he used the argon laser to make a rosette pattern on the footplate, to create a fenestra slightly larger than 0.6 mm in diameter. Analysis of the audiological results of the two groups, showed no differences at six or twelve months. Surgery was performed under local anaesthesia, but no patients experienced any vertigo during the application of the laser energy. The laser was useful in controlling bleeding around the oval window. McGee concludes that laser stapedotomy 'causes very little trauma and a minimum of physiological disturbance', but estimates that a follow up of some four to five years will be needed to assess whether the laser stapedotomy actually confers any benefit.

The use of the laser in otology

Whilst the results above show that the laser may be used safely to create a fenestra in the footplate, they fail to show any benefit of the laser over conventional techniques. The good results obtained are likely to be a reflection of the surgical skills of the surgeons involved rather than any intrinsic quality of the laser, although Perkins points out that the laser does allow one to deal with the problem of the floating footplate much more easily than would usually be the case. Di Bartolomeo found the laser useful in dealing with an obliterative footplate, but McGee found that in such cases the bone became too hot and felt that the use of a cutting burr was safer and more efficient. Thus even if the laser is used the high levels of skill in conventional techniques need to be maintained.

8.5 Acoustic neuroma

The laser has been used to facilitate the removal of tumours at the cerebellopontine angle. Glasscock, Jackson and Whitaker (1981) used the argon laser to debulk the tumour mass, and were able to do so without excessive pulling and tugging of surrounding structures. Similarly, if a piece of tumour remained attached to cranial nerves, major blood vessels or the brain stem, it could be vaporized with a minimum of trauma. A similar report of the usefulness of the laser in rapidly reducing the tumour mass was given by Gardner, Robertson and Clark (1983) although in this series a CO_2 laser was used.

8.6 Conclusions

Despite the fears that the use of the laser might cause irreversible damage to the labyrinth if it were used in the middle ear, the clinical reports which have been published so far would seem to indicate that the laser may be used safely in the field of otology. What has not been determined is whether the laser confers any real advantage over conventional techniques. From a review of the current literature it would seem that the only situation where the laser offers real benefits is in surgery performed around the oval window, when in particular, work may be carried out on the stapes whilst ensuring that no traumatic movement is transmitted to the inner ear. Thus it may be helpful in cases of chronic suppurative otitis media and in stapedectomy surgery – especially in cases of a floating footplate.

In a world where there are no financial restraints, then any otologist would possess a laser as part of his surgical equipment, but in these days of financial constraint then one has seriously to question whether the considerable expenses involved could not be put to better use.

References

Di Bartolomeo, J. R. and Ellis, M. (1980), The Argon laser in otology. *Laryngoscope*, **90**, 1786–96.
Escudero, L. H., Castro, A. O., Drumond, M., Porto, S. P. S., Bozinis, D. G., Penna, A. F. S. and Gallego-Lluesma, E. (1979), Argon laser in human tympanoplasty. *Arch. Otolaryngol.*, **105**, 252–3.
Fox, J. L., Stein, M. N., Hayes, J. R. and Green, R. C. (1968), Effects of laser irradiation on the central nervous system. The intracranial explosion. *J. Neurol. Neurosurg. Psychiat.*, **31**, 43–9.
Gantz, B. J., Jenkins, H. A., Kishimoto, S. and Fisch, U. (1982), Argon laser stapedotomy. *Ann. Otol.*, **91**, 25–6.
Gardner, G., Robertson, J. H. and Clark, W. C. (1983), 105 patients operated upon for cerebellopontine angle tumours – experience using combined approach and Carbon Dioxide laser. *Laryngoscope*, **93**, 1049–55.
Glasscock, M. E., Jackson, C. G. and Whitaker, S. R. (1981), The Argon laser in acoustic tumour surgery. *Laryngoscope*, **91**, 1405–16.
Goode, R. L. Carbon Dioxide laser myringotomy. *Laryngoscope*, **92**, 420–3.
Keleman, G., Laor, Y. and Klein, E. (1967), Laser induced ear damage. *Arch. Otolaryngol.*, **86**, 21–7.
Lipman, S., Zimm, E., Maloney, R., Guelcher, R. and Anon, J. (1987), Carbon Dioxide laser myringotomy. *Lasers Surg. Med.*, **7**, 99.
McGee, T. M. (1983), The Argon laser in surgery for chronic ear disease and otosclerosis. *Laryngoscope*, **93**, 1177–82.
Palva, T. (1982), Obliteration of the mastoid cavity and reconstruction of the canal wall. *Otolaryngology, Butterworths International Medical Review I. Otology*. Butterworths, London.
Perkins, R. C. (1980), Laser stapedotomy for otosclerosis. *Laryngoscope*, **90**, 228–40.
Ricci, T. and Mazzoni, M. (1985), Experimental investigation of temperature gradients in the inner ear following Argon laser exposure. *J. Laryngol. Otol.*, **99**, 359–62.
Sataloff, J. (1967), Experimental use of the laser in otosclerotic stapes. *Arch. Otolaryngol*, **85**, 614–16.
Stahle, J. and Hogberg, L. (1965), Laser and the labyrinthe. Some preliminary experiments on pigeons. *Acta Otolaryngol*, **60**, 367–73.
Stahle, J., Hogberg, L. and Engstrom, B. (1972), The laser as a tool in inner ear surgery. *Acta Otolaryngol.*, **73**, 27–37.
Thoma, J., Unger, V. and Kastenbauer, E. (1981), Temperatur und druckmessungen im innen ohr bei der Anwendung der Argon lasers. *Laryngol. Rhinol. Otol.* (Stutts), **60**, 587–90.
Thoma, J., Mrowinski, D. and Kastenbauer, E. R. (1986), Experimental investigations on the suitability of the Carbon Dioxide laser for stapedotomy. *Ann. Otol. Rhinol. Laryngol.*, **95**, 126–31.
Wilpizeski, C., Sataloff, J., Doyle, J. and Behrendt, T. (1972), Selective vestibular ablation in monkeys by laser irradiation. *Laryngoscope*, **82**, 1045–58.

9 Photodynamic therapy

J. A. S. CARRUTH

The concept of tumour destruction by photoactivation of a sensitizer began with the observation by Raab (1900) that exposure to light killed *Paramoecium* which had been sensitized with an acridine dye.

The technique is now being extensively researched, both in the laboratory and in increasingly well-constructed clinical trials, and when it is fully developed it should represent an important modality for the treatment of many forms of localized malignant disease.

In an ideal form, a patient with a malignant tumour is given a photosensitive tumour sensitizer which produces minimal side effects and which is selectively absorbed or retained by malignant tissues, giving a high tumour/normal tissue ratio. This sensitizer should be photoactivated by light at a wavelength which provides adequate tissue penetration, and when activated should cause the release of a toxic substance or substances which will destroy the tumour, leaving surrounding normal tissues undamaged.

The current situation using red light and haematoporphyrin derivative (HPD) begins to approach the ideal, but it appears certain that developments under investigation will result in significant improvements in the technique. However, it will be several years before another light/sensitizer combination will be developed to a state where clinical trials will be appropriate.

9.1 Tumour sensitizer

From the observations by Policard (1924), who noticed that certain tumours exhibited fluorescence and attributed this to an accumulation of endogenous porphyrins, much of the research into tumour sensitizers has been on the porphyrins.

Schwartz first produced haematoporphyrin derivative by treating haematoporphyrin with a mixture of acetic and sulphuric acids, fol-

Photodynamic therapy

lowed by hydrolysis under basic conditions. Its use as a tumour localizer was first described by Lipson, Baldes and Olsen (1961) who showed a close correlation between tumour fluorescence and malignant histology. This same group also carried out a small amount of clinical work.

Since that time a considerable amount of research on this substance has been carried out, much of it by Dr Tom Dougherty and his co-workers at Roswell Park Memorial Institute in Buffalo, New York. From research carried out to date, it became apparent that it was appropriate to begin clinical trials but, of course, it is also evident that further laboratory studies are needed to establish the technique on a firm scientific footing.

9.1.1 CHEMISTRY

Haematoporphyrin derivative is a mixture of porphyrins, and Dougherty, Potter and Weishaupt (1983) have identified the active component as dihaematoporphyrin ether (DHE) and this is now used in many of the clinical studies marketed as Photofrin 2. However, other chemists believe that further work on the identification of the active component is appropriate and other substances have already been suggested, including dihaematoporphyrin ester.

Other sensitizers have been and are being extensively researched. Uroporphyrin I was identified by El Far and Pimstone (1981) as an 'ideal sensitizer' but other workers have not confirmed their results.

A significant amount of research is being carried out on a wide range of phthalocyanines which are pure substances that can be synthesized and appear to offer great promise.

It appears certain that other compounds will be identified and used as superior tumour sensitizers and it is to be hoped that a sensitizer will be found which is activated at a low infrared wavelength as this provides optimal tissue penetration.

9.1.2 TISSUE DISTRIBUTION

Using an autoradiographic technique, Bugelski, Potter and Dougherty (1981) showed that HPD is at first widely distributed throughout the body and is then selectively retained by malignant tissues. However, it has been suggested from quantitative fluorescence studies that HPD may be selectively absorbed by malignant tissues.

The mechanism for this retention remains uncertain, but it is thought to be related to the abnormal tumour circulation. Within tumour tissue HPD is distributed in a ratio of 5:1 in stroma/cells.

There is also significant retention in other normal tissues including liver, spleen, kidneys and skin. The retention of HPD in skin accounts for the severe skin photosensitization which occurs for 3–4 weeks after injection.

9.1.3 MODE OF ACTION

It has been shown by Weishaupt, Gomer and Dougherty (1976) that when HPD is photoactivated, singlet oxygen is produced by energy transfer from the excited porphyrin molecule. This highly reactive, transient state of the oxygen molecule is cytotoxic by oxidizing sensitive bonds.

It has been shown that oxygen is necessary for this reaction, but it has also been suggested that in the absence of oxygen, other cytotoxic mechanisms may be responsible for tumour destruction.

9.1.4 SITE OF ACTION

It appears that there is photodynamic activity, both within the vascular stroma and at a cellular level. At a cellular level Coppola *et al.* (1980) and Moan *et al.* (1982) have shown that changes *in vitro* first occur in the cell around the mitochondria and damage also occurs to the cell membrane. However, Henderson and Dougherty (1983) have studied cell survival after PDT and have shown that cell death occurs rapidly and progressively from 1 to 10 hours after photoactivation, but that immediately after PDT no tumour cell inactivation was found. They concluded that this pattern of cell death was exactly similar to that which occurred after cutting off the circulation to the tumour, and that the majority of photodynamic activity occurred in the vascular stroma.

9.1.5 ADMINISTRATION OF SENSITIZER

At present, HPD is given by slow intravenous injection in a dose of 3 mg/kg body weight or 1.5–2 mg/kg of DHE. No significant side effects have been reported from the injection.

Research is in progress on the local administration of the sensitizer, either by injection or by local application through skin or mucosa.

9.1.6 SIDE EFFECTS

The only significant side effect which has been reported is severe skin photosensitization which lasts for 3–4 weeks after the injection. A number of techniques have been used in an attempt to overcome this problem, which many patients find distressing, but no technique has

Photodynamic therapy

given uniformly successful results, and this side effect remains the only significant clinical problem with the technique of photodynamic therapy.

9.2 Light sources

HPD is best activated by blue light, but this provides inadequate tissue penetration and it could not, therefore, be used to treat tumours except those of only a few millimetres in thickness.

The wavelength which has been identified as the 'optimal compromise' is 630 nm which activates HPD and provides adequate tissue penetration.

At first, a wide range of light sources using both filtered and unfiltered light were used for PDT, but it became apparent that to produce adequate power levels of monochromatic light which could be transmitted via a flexible fibre, a laser was the optimal light source.

Lasers are, therefore, somewhat peripheral to photodynamic therapy, but the technique has been 'adopted' by a number of national and international laser societies and this chapter therefore appears relevant to this volume.

Much of the work has been carried out with a tuneable dye laser in which an argon laser drives the dye laser, which usually uses a rhodamine dye. The advantage of this system is that the wavelength can be tuned over a significant range of the visible spectrum using a range of dyes, and a birefringent crystal. This means that a wavelength could be selected to activate other sensitizers which may be developed in the future, but the power level available is, at best, only 25% of that of the driving argon laser.

Recently, work has begun with the pulsed gold vapour laser and this has been compared with the dye laser by McKenzie and Carruth (1986). The gold vapour laser produces pulsed red light at a wavelength of 627.8 nm and it has been suggested that this pulsed beam may penetrate better into tissues than the continuous wave dye laser beam. However, further research has failed to confirm this initial impression.

High power levels are available with this laser allowing large tumours to be treated rapidly, but the wavelength is fixed and it could not, therefore, be used to activate other sensitizers. However, it is relatively simple to change the metal in the laser tube to copper and this copper vapour laser could then be used to drive a tuneable dye laser.

9.2.1 DELIVERY SYSTEMS

Using a glass fibre delivery system, it has been shown that with surface irradiation red light at 630 nm penetrates to a depth of 5–10 mm depending on the nature of the tissue and on tissue homogeneity.

Clinical studies

Fibres with diffusing bulb tips can be used to photoirradiate the whole of the inside of a hollow viscus, such as the bladder, and fibres with diffusing cylinder tips can be used to irradiate circumferential tumours of the oesophagus and tracheobronchial tree, and these may also be implanted into more bulky tumours to destroy cylinders of tumour.

9.3 Animal studies

It has been shown that a wide range of tumours, both induced and naturally occurring, can be ablated by the technique of PDT using HPD or DHE and red light. However, a lesser amount of information is available on the effects of PDT on normal tissues and many studies in this area are in progress and are essential before PDT can be widely accepted and used clinically. In addition, research is in progress on the interrelationship between PDT and radiotherapy and between PDT and hyperthermia.

9.4 Clinical studies

9.4.1 DIAGNOSTIC

When exposed to violet light, tumour containing HPD exhibits a red fluorescence which can be utilized in the diagnosis of malignant or grossly dysplastic lesions and is particularly relevant in identifying small tumours and malignant foci in multifocal disease.

A considerable amount of interest has been shown in the identification of early pre-invasive lung carcinoma by the technique of fluorescent bronchoscopy. Using essentially similar equipment, three groups of workers in the USA and Japan (Kinsey, Cortese and Sanderson, (1978); Balchum *et al.* (1982); and Hayata *et al.* (1982)) have been able to detect small lesions of the tracheobronchial tree with great accuracy and much more rapidly than has been possible using a standard 'white light' bronchoscopic technique. The equipment described consisted of a blue-light-enhanced fibreoptic bronchoscope with a krypton laser to produce the violet light and an image intensifier to detect the areas of faint fluorescence.

Another area in which tumour fluorescence has been shown to be of value is in the identification of malignant foci in multifocal disease of the bladder.

It has been suggested that tumour fluorescence may be of significant value in the identification of malignant areas in widespread dysplasia of

Photodynamic therapy

the oral cavity but although the idea has great potential, this has not yet been realized in clinical studies.

9.4.2 TREATMENT TECHNIQUE

A majority of clinical studies employ an essentially similar technique. On day 1 the patient is given HPD or DHE in an appropriate dose by slow intravenous injection. Patients are then warned about the skin photosensitization and how to avoid sunburn.

After 72 hours the tumour is photoirradiated using a fibreoptic delivery system with an appropriate fibre tip for the lesion. The treatment power (mW/cm^2) will obviously depend on the power of the laser and the area to be treated, and it has been suggested that a minimum treatment power of approximately 10 mW/cm^2 may be necessary for photodynamic therapy. However, other workers, particularly in the field of bladder disease, have shown that a photodynamic response can be obtained with much lower power levels. If a fibre or fibres are implanted into the tumour, a dose of 500 mW/cm implanted fibre is often used.

Whatever the treatment power the total dose appears to be the most important measurement (J/cm^2). The doses used remain somewhat empirical and are based on current clinical impressions rather than hard data. For subcutaneous nodular disease of the chest wall, a total dose of 25/cm^2 should cause tumour destruction with preservation of the overlying skin. For ulcerated lesions a dose of 100–200 J/cm^2 is used to provide maximal tumour necrosis.

With some of the high power levels, particularly when the beam is focused by the eye onto retinal tumours, there is undoubtedly a significant hyperthermic effect.

9.4.3 TRIALS

A number of clinical trials, some controlled, but most uncontrolled, have been and are being performed. Many of the early studies remain anecdotal but the quality of trial design is improving rapidly, and the role of PDT should soon be established on a scientific basis.

Subcutaneous nodular disease from carcinoma of the breast has been most widely studied and Dougherty (unpublished report) has estimated that in 60–80% of patients, local tumour control can be achieved.

Studies on carcinoma in situ of the bladder, which has failed conventional treatment, are being reported with light diffused to the whole of the inside of the bladder by a bulb on the delivery fibre, a diffusing medium in the bladder or a mechanical device. This field represents one of the most exciting and valuable areas for PDT, as the alternative in uncontrolled disease is a cystectomy. Some very encouraging early results have been achieved.

Lung tumours have been treated for palliation when a major airway has been obstructed by tumour and trials are in progress to compare PDT with thermal tumour ablation using the Nd-YAG laser. Some early lung tumours have been treated for cure when resection has been contraindicated or refused, and some long-term tumour controls have been reported.

The role of PDT in tumours of the eye and of the brain is being evaluated.

PDT can be used to treat basal cell carcinoma of the skin when all other modalities have failed, or when further radiotherapy or wide resection are inappropriate. Excellent results can be obtained and it has been suggested that PDT may become the treatment of choice for multiple basal cell carcinomas as these are extremely difficult to manage by conventional techniques.

In addition, lesions of Bowen's disease can be ablated rapidly and successfully. In the author's unpublished series, two patients with more than 700 lesions were treated resulting in complete tumour regression.

9.4.4 HEAD AND NECK

Tumours of the head and neck are very appropriate for treatment with this modality as they are accessible, relatively small and remain localized. Surgery is always mutilating to some extent, either to the appearance of the patient or his ability to talk or swallow, and it may be inappropriate or refused by the patient.

One major series has been reported to date by Wile et al. (1982, 1984). In this on-going series all patients had failed all other modalities of treatment and 114 sites were treated in 39 patients with a complete response in 28 and partial response (reduction of tumour by more than 50%) in 42. There have been several long remissions of more than one year, and tumours of the tongue appeared to be particularly sensitive to this form of treatment.

In the author's series (Carruth and McKenzie 1985), a number of patients with adenoid cystic carcinoma of the maxilla following radical surgery and of the post-nasal space have been treated and control has been achieved. However, it is not possible to claim a cure with this tumour which is notorious for recurrence after a period of many years.

9.5 Conclusion

The technique of PDT remains to be fully evaluated and undoubtedly

Photodynamic therapy

new sensitizers will be developed in the future. However, even in its present form it offers considerable potential for the management of many forms of localized malignant disease.

References

Balchum, O. J., Doiron, D. R., Profio, A. E. and Huth, G. C. (1982), Fluorescence bronchoscopy for localizing early bronchial cancer and carcinoma in situ. In *Recent Results in Cancer Research*, Springer-Verlag, Berlin, pp. 97–120.

Bugelski, P. J., Potter, C. W. and Dougherty, T. J. (1981), Autoradiographic distribution of hematoporphyrin derivative in normal and tumour tissue of the mouse. *Cancer Res.*, **41**, 4606–12.

Carruth, J. A. S. and McKenzie, A. L. (1985), Preliminary report of a pilot study of photoradiation therapy for the treatment of superficial malignancies of the skin, head and neck. *Eur. J. Surg. Oncol.*, **11**, 47–50.

Coppola, A., Viggiani, E., Salzarulo, L. and Rasile, G. (1980), Ultra-structural changes in lymphoma cells treated with haematoporphyrin and light. *Am. J. Pathol.*, **99**, 175.

Dougherty, T. J., Potter, W. R. and Weishaupt, K. R. (1983), The structure of the active component of hematoporphyrin derivative. In *Porphyrins in Tumour Phototherapy*, (eds A. Andreoni and R. Cubeddu), Plenum Press, New York, pp. 22–35.

El-Far, M. A. and Pimstone, N. R. (1981), Superiority of Uroporphyrin I over other porphyrins in selective tumour localization. In *Proceedings of the Clayton Foundation Symposium on Porphyrin Localization and Treatment of Tumours*, Santa Barbara, California.

Hayata, Y., Kato, H., Konaka, C., Ono, J., Matsushima, Y. and Nishimiya, K. (1982), Fibreoptic bronchoscopic laser photoradiation for tumour localization in lung cancer. *Chest*, **82**, 10–14.

Henderson, B. W. and Dougherty, T. J. (1983), Studies on the mechanism of tumour destruction by photoradiation therapy (PRT), in *Proceedings of the Clayton Foundation Symposium on Porphyrin Localization and Treatment of Tumours*, Santa Barbara, California.

Kinsey, J. H., Cortese, D. A. and Sanderson, D. R. (1978), Detection of hematoporphyrin fluorescence during fibreoptic bronchoscopy to localize early bronchogenic carcinoma. *Mayo Clin. Proc.*, **53**, 594–600.

Lipson, R. L., Baldes, E. J. and Olsen, A. M. (1961), Haematoporphyrin derivative: A new aid for endoscopic detection of malignant disease. *J. Thorac. Cardiovasc. Surg.*, **42**, 623–9.

McKenzie, A. L. and Carruth, J. A. S. (1986), A comparison of gold-vapour and dye lasers for photodynamic therapy. *Lasers Med. Sci.*, **1**, 117.

Moan, J., Johannessen, J. W., Christensen, T., Espevik, T. and McGhie, J. B. (1982), Porphyrin-sensitized photoinactivation of human cells *in vitro*. *Am. J. Pathol.*, **109**, 184–92.

Policard, A. (1924), Etudes sur les aspects offerts par des tumeur experimentales examinée à la lumiere de woods. *C.R. Soc. Biol.*, **91**, 1423–4.

Raab, O. (1900), Uber die wirkung floureszirenden stoffe auf infusoria. *Z. Biol.*, **39**, 524.

References

Weishaupt, K. R., Gomer, C. J. and Dougherty, T. J. (1976), Identification of singlet oxygen as the cytotoxic agent in photo-inactivation of a murine tumour. *Cancer Res.*, **36**, 2326–9.

Wile, A. G., Coffey, J., Nahobedion, M. Y., Baghdassarian, R., Mason, G. R. and Berns, M. W. (1984), Laser photoradiation therapy of cancer. An update of the experience at the University of California, Irvine. *Lasers Surg. Med.*, **4**, 5–12.

Wile, A. G., Dahlman, A., Burns, R. G. and Berns, M .W. (1982), Laser photoradiation therapy of cancer following hematoporphyrin sensitization. *Lasers Surg. Med.*, **2**, 163–8.

Index

Page numbers in *italics* refer to figures

Acoustic neuroma 164
Adenoid cystic carcinoma of maxilla 173
Adenoma, pleomorphic, of palate 116–18
Aiming lasers 26–7
Amyloid
  localized tumours 72
  tracheobronchial 95
Anaesthesia, CO_2 laser surgery 35–44
  adult patients 35, 37–43
  complications 36–7
  endotracheal tubes *see* Endotracheal tubes
  laryngeal disease 48
  mouth lesions 43
  paediatric patients 44
  surgical requirements 35
  surgical stimulus 35
  tracheostomy patient 43
Anterior skull base tumours 155
Argon laser 12–13
  eye protection 28
  laser-tissue interaction 23–4
  nasal surgery 148–9, 151
Arytenoidectomy 71–2
Atelectasis, post-endoscopic laser surgery 98

Basal cell carcinoma of skin 173
Beam parallelism 1–4
Bladder carcinoma 172
Bowen's disease 173
Brain tumours 173
Breast carcinoma 172
Bronchoscopes 90
  ventilating *91*

Candidiasis, chronic hyperplastic (candidal leukoplakia) 120
  follow up 122–4
  management 121–4
Carbon dioxide laser xi–xii, 6–12
  absorption coefficient 21
  anaesthesia *see* Anaesthesia
  coupler *89*
  eye protection 28
  laser-tissue interaction 21
    subsurface damage 21–2
  nasal surgery 147–8; *see also* Nasal surgery
  original endoscopic delivery system *88*
  power variation 11
  principles of operation 7–9
  technology 9–12
  tracheobronchial tree *see* Tracheobronchial tree
Carcinogenesis 72–3
Carcinoma *in situ* (erythroplakia) 73–5
Carcinoma of larynx *see* Laryngeal carcinoma
Cardiac arryhthmias, post-endoscopic laser surgery 54, 97
Choanal atresia 154
Chondroma, tracheobronchial 95
Classification of CW lasers 26–7
Contact ulcer 61
Copper tubing 42
Crow–Davis mouth-gag 49

Dedo laryngoscope 48
Denture-induced hyperplasia 115–16
Dexamethasone 54, 66
Dihaematoporphyrin ether 168
Dingman mouth-gag 49
Dye laser 7, 15–16, 99
  gold vapour laser compared 170

177

Index

Ear *see* Otology
Endotracheal tubes 39–43
 none used 41–3
 non-inflammable plastic 41
 Norton and De Vos 39, 41, 52
 protection 37–9, 52, 53
 PVC compared with red rubber 37
Enflurane 44
ENT lasers, specific 6–18
Ethmoidal tumours 155
Extended source exposure 25–6
External auditory meatus 160
External ear 160
Eye
 laser damage 25–6
 protection 27–8
 tumours 173

Fire hazard 51, 52–3

Glottic web 67–8
Gold vapour laser 6, 7, 16–18, 170
 dye laser compared 170
Granulomas, laryngeal 59–61
 intubation 59, 61
 prevention 61

Haemangioma
 capillary 66–7
 cavernous 66–7
 tracheobronchial 95
Haematoporphin derivative (HPD) xii, 15, 19, 99, 167–8
 administration 169
 chemistry 168
 light sources 170
 mode of action 169
 side effects 169–70
 site of action 169
 tissue distribution 168–9
 see also Photodynamic therapy
Halothane 44
Hemiglossectomy *125–7*
 anterior partial 126–7
He-Ne laser beam, red 3–4, 6
Hereditary haemorrhagic telangectasia 149, 153
Hopkins Rod Telescopes 90, *92*
Hyperkeratosis papilloma (papillary keratosis) 73
Hypopharyngeal diverticulum
 aetiology 133–4

carcinoma 134
diagnosis 134
familial incidence 133–4
microendoscopic treatment 135–8
 complications 137, 140, 142, 144
 electrocoagulation 138
 methods 138–42
 patients 138–42
 results 142–4
myotomy of cricopharyngeus 136, 137
myotomy of sphincter 135
surgical excision 134–5
symptoms 134
triangle of Killian 133, 135

Infra red coherent laser beam xii
Intrabeam exposure 25–6
Irradiance (power density) 18, 19, 25

Jackson–Boyce sniffing position 50
Jako–Kleinsasser laryngoscopes 48
Jet ventilation 41

Keratosis 73, *74*
 papillary (hyperkeratosis papilloma) 73
 treatment 133, 135
Killian's triangle 133, 135

Laryngeal carcinoma 76–84
 airway preservation 83
 current treatment plans 84
 cytoreduction (debulking) 83–4
 diagnosis 76
 epidermoid *82–3*
 excision biopsy: cure 76–7
 staging 77
 recurrent, after radiation therapy 77–81
 verrucous *78–9*
Laryngeal disease 47–85
 anaesthesia 48; *see also* Anaesthesia
 exposure of operating field 48–50
 instruments 50–1
 magnification 50
 postoperative care 53–4
 safety procedures 51–3
 time provision 50
Laryngeal sarcoma *80–1*
Laryngeal stenosis 67–71
 glottic webb 67–8

178

Index

laser surgery 71
  posterior glottic 68
  subglottic 68–9, 70–1
  supraglottic 67
  synechiae 67–8
Laryngocoele 65–6
Laser Controlled Area 30
Laser, derivation of word 3
Laser physics 1–6
  beam parallelism 1–4
  population inversion 4–6
  spontaneous emission 2
  stimulated emission 1–3
Laser Protection Adviser 29, 30
Laser Protection Supervisor 29, 30
Laser safety 24–31
  accidental exposure 24
  classification of CW lasers 26–7
  extended-source exposure 25–6
  eye 25–6
    protection 27–8
  intrabeam exposure 25–6
  maximum permissible exposure 26
  organization 28–9
  reflections 24–5
  safety codes 29–30
Laser–tissue interaction 19–24
  argon laser 23–4
  CO_2 laser radiation 21
    subsurface damage 21–2
  Nd-YAG laser 22–3
  thermal effects 19–21
    burning 20
    coagulation 20
    vaporization 20
Leukoplakia, oral 106, 107, 120, 122
  follow up 122–4
Lewy–Kleinsasser systems 49–50
Lichen planus, oral 120–1
  follow up 121–2
  management 122–4
Light amplification by stimulated emission of radiation (laser) 3
Lung tumours 173
Lymphangiomas 72
Lynch suspension system 48

Maxillary adenoid cystic carcinoma 173
Maximum permissible exposure 26–7
Micromanipulator 11
Middle ear 161–2

Mouth lesions see Oral lesions
Mucous cyst, oral 116
Myringotomy 161–2

Nasal septum 148
Nasal surgery 147–55
  anterior nasal space 153–4
  argon laser 148–9, 151
  CO_2 laser 147–8
    technique 149–51
  external nose 152
  Nd-YAG laser 149
  paranasal sinuses 154–5
  posterior nasal space 153–4
Neodymium-YAG laser 13–14
  experimental otology 158, 159
  filtering glasses in goggles 52
  for haemangioma 66–7
  laser-tissue interaction 22–3
  nasal surgery 149
Neurofibromas 72
Norton and De Vos endotracheal tube 39, 41, 52

Oral cavity, CO_2 laser surgery in 101–30
  advantages 102
  alternative surgical techniques 101–2
  anaesthesia 43, 114; see also Anaesthesia
  benign lesions 43, 118
  chronic hyperplastic candidiasis (candidal leukoplakia) 120
    follow up 122–4
    management 122–4
  complications
    early postoperative 128–9
    immediate 128
    late postoperative 129–30
  denture-induced hyperplasia 115–16
  distribution of lesions 113
  granuloma following 129, 130
  healing of mucosal wounds 109–13
    biological aspects 110–13
    clinical aspects 109–10
  laser variables 103–6
    duration of exposure 106
    power density 105–6
    spot size 104–5

179

Index

Oral cavity (*contd*)
 leukoplakia *see* Leukoplakia
 malignant lesions 124–8
  indications 126–8
  reconstruction 126–8
  surgical technique 124–6
 mucous cyst 116
 histology of lesions 114
 pleomorphic adenoma 116–18
 premalignant lesions 118–24
  follow up 122–4
  management 121–2
 ranula 116
 tissue variables 107–9
  accessibility 107
  depth of lesion 108
  excision or vaporization? 108
  site 107
  size of lesion 108
  tissue surface 108
  veloglossal incompetence following 130
Osteochondroma obstructing bronchus 92
Otitis media
 chronic suppurative 162–3
 secretory 161
Otology 157–64
 acoustic neuroma 164
 clinical applications 160
 experimental background 157–60
 external auditory meatus 160
 external ear 160
 middle ear 161–2
 otitis media
  chronic suppurative 162–3
  secretory 161
 otosclerosis 163–4
 stapedectomy 163–4
 tympanic membrane 161–2
 tympanoplasty 162
Otosclerosis 163–4

Palatal pleomorphic adenoma 116–18
Papillary keratosis (hyperkeratosis papilloma) 73
Papilloma 62
 hyperkeratotic 65
 keratinizing 64–5
Papova viruses 62
Paranasal sinuses 154–5

Peristomal granulation, tracheobronchial 95
Photodynamic therapy xii–xiii, 167–74
 clinical studies 171–3
 delivery systems 170–1
 diagnostic studies 171–2
 eye protection 28
 head and neck tumours 173
 treatment technique 172
 trials 172–3
 see also Haematoporphyrin derivate
Photofrin 2 168
Photon 2–3, 4
Phthalocyanines 168
Pilling–Boston University system *49*, 50
Pleomorphic adenoma of palate 116–18
Polypoid vocal fold lesions 55–8
Population inversion 4–6
Port wine stain of nose 152
Post-rhinoplasty red nose 152
Power density (irradiance) 18, 19, 25
Premalignant disease, laryngeal 73–5
Propofol 41

Ranula 116
Recurrent respiratory papillomatosis 62–4, 95
 treatment plan 64
Red nose, post-rhinoplasty 152
Rhinophyma 152
Ruby laser 157, 158

Safety codes 29–30
Sanders injector 41, 42, 44
Sarcoidosis, tracheobronchial 95
Sarcoma of larynx *80–1*
Silicon endotracheal tube 39–41
Spontaneous emission 2
Spot sizes 11, 18–19
Stapedectomy 163–4
Stapes footplate, laser effects on 159–60
Stimulated emission 1–3
Suction devices xiii, 51
Surgical emphysema 41, 44
Synechiae, laryngeal 67–8

Telangectasia 152
 hereditary haemorrhagic 149, 163
Tolidine blue 0 dye, 51, 73, 75, 76

Index

Tongue, carcinoma of *125–7*
  see also Hemiglossectomy
tracheal stenosis with Tracheomalacia 96
Tracheobronchial tree, endoscopic laser surgery 87–99
  CO_2 laser system 87–91, 98–9
    anaesthesia 88, 90
    indications 95–6
    soft tissue interaction 94–5
  complications 97–8
  contraindications 96
  indications 95–6
  Nd-YAG 93–4, 98–9
    soft tissue interaction 94–5
  post-operative evaluation 96–7
  pre-operative evaluation 96–7
Tracheobronchial wall perforations 97
Tracheomalacia, with tracheal stenosis 96

Triangle of Killian 133, 135
Tumour sensitizer 167–8
Tympanic membrane 161–2
Tympanoplasty 162

Uroporphyrin I 168

Vasomotor rhinitis 149, 154
Venturi ventilation 63, 66
Vidian neurectomy 154
Viral papilloma 44
Vocal cord abductor paralysis, bilateral 71–2
Vocal fold
  cysts 59, *60*
  polypoid lesions 55–8
  polyps 58–9
Vocal nodules 54–5
Voice rest 53–4